Take Care of Ivan

*...a caregiver's struggle to
save her husband*

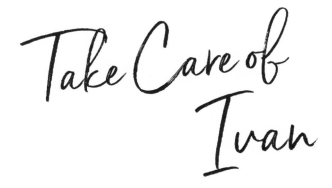

Take Care of Ivan

*...a caregiver's struggle to
save her husband*

SUZANNE ANEST

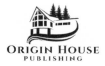

ORIGIN HOUSE
PUBLISHING

Take Care of Ivan: A Caregiver's Struggle to Save her Husband

Published by ORIGIN HOUSE PUBLISHING
SHADY COVE, OREGON

Library of Congress Control Number: 2019903822

ANEST, SUZANNE, Author
TAKE CARE OF IVAN
SUZANNE ANEST

ISBN: 978-0-578-47901-9

MEDICAL / Caregiving
FAMILY & RELATIONSHIPS / Death, Grief, Bereavement

Editing by Donna Mazzitelli, The Word Heartiste
Cover Design by Donna Cunningham of BeauxArts.Design
Interior Design by Deanna Estes of Lotus Design, LLC

QUANTITY PURCHASES: Schools, companies, professional groups, clubs, and other organizations may qualify for special terms when ordering quantities of this title. For information, email Info@OriginHousePublishing.com.

When angels visit us,
we do not hear the rustle of wings,
nor feel the feathery touch
of the breast of a dove;
but we know their presence
By the love they create in our hearts.

Mary Baker Eddy – Angels

To Ivan H. Jester,
a strong man who lived this story
from another viewpoint.

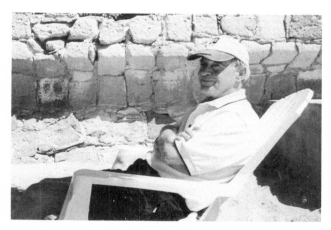

Ivan – 1997

Table of Contents

The Journey to March

Moving Forward...Walking Backward

Epilogue

Some Final Thoughts for Caregivers

Acknowledgments

About The Author

Introduction

My story involves cancer, but cancer is just one of many life-threatening conditions that impact people's lives. When a serious illness occurs to someone you know, it not only impacts that person, but it impacts everyone who is connected to that person, especially the caregiver. The way it impacts each person, patient, or caregiver is based on their personal background, childhood, past experiences, and beliefs. However, no matter how unique each person's story may be regarding the illness, the feelings of one caregiver to another are remarkably similar.

Many of us have been taught that the meaning of love includes sacrifice, suffering, and maybe even martyrdom. What we come to believe about what it means to take care of another person includes all of the "shoulds" and expectations from others, as well as our own self-imposed expectations: to never complain or admit to struggling with the caregiver role.

When I became a primary caregiver, I believed I needed to be strong, to put on a game face, and to be a great daughter, mother, wife, and friend. I carried the burden of ensuring the health and well-being of my husband, and I was frequently plagued with feelings of guilt and a sense of inadequacy, especially when things weren't working out the way we had hoped. I often felt that I was responsible for what was going wrong.

I was fifty-one years old when my husband became ill, the youngest of four children in a family that believed in hard work and a strong sense of responsibility. I did not have a college education, like my other three siblings, because I had married and begun full-time work at the age of eighteen. My father passed away when I was twenty-one, and I had been married and divorced twice before marrying Ivan at the age of twenty-nine.

I had entered the healthcare field in 1974, and for over thirty years, I sold employee benefits that also involved managing medical claims. I strove to prove myself as a successful businesswoman in an industry that was male-dominated, and I considered myself a strong woman who was knowledgeable about the healthcare industry. I had also learned to be a fighter. Above all else, I'd become a self-made woman who was results-oriented but continually battled a fear of failure and a sense of inadequacy.

When the time came to care for my husband, I thought my determination and positive attitude would provide the emotional strength I needed as a caregiver. I also thought my background in the medical field would serve me well. Dealing with cancer changed all that, and going through it all as a caregiver changed me. I soon realized I had no idea how the medical profession operated and that my background, which had been sprinkled with challenges and struggles, had not prepared me for the role of caregiver. I learned that the impact of my own background and experiences influenced how I viewed the events around me. I realized I wanted to control things that I had no control over.

Most of society has a view of what constitutes a "good person" versus a "bad person." We expect a person who is caring for someone else to say and do things that we believe are "good." We believe it is their duty. We typically don't expect a caregiver to express any thoughts or emotions of anger, frustration, or disgust toward the person who is ill. We attribute only loving and caring feelings to the caregiver. Yet, this distinction creates turmoil because feelings of anger, exhaustion, and even frustration with the ill occur frequently.

I experienced these thoughts and emotions and felt ashamed for having them. When they arose, I felt selfish or inadequate, so I didn't discuss or disclose these thoughts and feelings to anyone. I kept them inside, for fear of judgment or reprisal.

At the beginning of Ivan's diagnosis and treatment, I set up an email group that I referred to as the Health Watch Group. This distribution group initially consisted of our two daughters, who lived in California, and nine other friends and family members. I thought it would be easier to communicate through email since Ivan and I lived so far from everyone, but I had no idea about the impact and usefulness of this method of communication. As time passed, more and more people reached out to my daughter Alison or me and asked to be added to the distribution group. The communication allowed people to stay connected with the daily events without feeling that they were imposing on my time, but more importantly, these emails allowed me to detach and hide from personal contact with people, so I didn't have to reveal how I really felt about the scary moments that occurred.

I decided to retain these emails, intending to show Ivan what he had conquered in his journey to recovery once he was well again. The sequence of *Take Care of Ivan* is based on the many emails I printed and kept in a binder for him. I transcribed each of the emails I had sent to the group distribution and have entered them into this book, exactly as they were written. For that reason, you will see typographical errors and misspellings. They help to show how unimportant grammar was to me at the time they were written. The importance was to chronicle what was happening to Ivan.

They also provided a form of journaling for me and a memoir of the events I, too, was experiencing. They eventually served as a way to begin my personal healing, as I reread the challenges Ivan and I had gone through.

Take Care of Ivan is for any caregiver or family member who is dealing with a life-threatening illness or a progressive disease. My hope is that by reading my story, you will give yourself permission to accept and express yourself during your personal journey. My intention is that through my story, you may find hope and encouragement for your journey; that you will allow yourself to be there with love and compassion for yourself and everyone involved, including the person who is ill; and that you will recognize the influence of your background, childhood, and other personal experiences that preceded your caregiver role and set the stage for your emotional reactions, interpretations, and struggles. Finally, my deepest desire is that as you experience various events during your role as caregiver, with their many ups and downs, you will confide in someone about *all* your thoughts and feelings, including the negative ones, so that, above all else, your love and acceptance of yourself will prevail.

The Journey to March

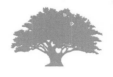

Chapter 1

Life with Ivan

I first met Ivan in 1979, at an open house for an insurance brokerage company in San Francisco. When he saw me enter the room, he was standing with a friend and commented to his friend that he had just seen the woman he was going to marry. Obviously, this was meant to be a joke; however, a year later, our paths crossed again.

I had a meeting with the hiring manager for a job opening at a different company, and that hiring manager turned out to be Ivan. At the time, I was going through my second divorce, and while I did not disclose the change in my marital status during the interview and subsequent employment, after the divorce was final, Ivan and I began to date. He was fourteen years older than me, and I was enamored with his financial drive, his dry sense of humor, and his love for me.

We were married in 1981, and I changed jobs to work for another insurance company since the company where we both worked did not allow both husband and wife to work at the same location. My daughter Alison was four years old at the time of our marriage, and Ivan adored her as if she were his own daughter.

In 1983, I gave birth to our daughter Sara, and after the traditional six weeks of staying home with my newborn, I returned to work in San Francisco. Ivan also continued to work in San Francisco, and although there were times when we commuted together for the one-hour drive into the city, the days were long, and I struggled to manage work, the household, and the needs of two children. Despite the challenges, I progressed in my sales career by achieving one of the top sales results for five years in a row.

By 1985, Ivan was having difficulty in his job, due to his heavy drinking and progressive alcoholism. While there were obvious signals when we dated and after we married, over time, his late nights of drinking increased. We began to fight about his constant drinking, so when his employer approached me with the request to join in an intervention about Ivan's drinking, I agreed.

We spent several weeks planning our surprise meeting with him. The intervention involved the Human Resources Department, his direct manager, one of his closest friends, and me. The plan was for each of us to express our concern about Ivan's drinking and state why it was having a negative impact, as well as to give him an ultimatum: that if he did not agree to stop drinking, he needed to enter a rehab center. It was especially frightening for me because I had to state that I would divorce him if he did not stop. While I wanted my husband back from the demons of alcohol that had pulled him away, I did not want another failed marriage. I worried that Ivan would not agree to stop and my life would be a failure again. The fact that the meeting was also a secret until we could confront him added stress to the days that preceded our meeting.

A few days before the planned meeting, the employer approached me once again and informed me that they had misgivings about the company's role in the meeting. They wanted to abort the plan, due to legal concerns. I was furious and heartbroken at the same time. As I openly cried in front of the human resources vice president, I told him we needed to move forward with the plan. I told him that they had started this plan of action, and I would not allow them to back out. They stared at me for a moment and then agreed to proceed. I had successfully placed the nail in my husband's coffin with work, friendship, and marriage if he did not agree to the ultimatum. I felt empty and scared, but I also knew I needed to be strong. I believed that Ivan would waiver or not agree to the conditions if he saw any sign of weakness in any one of us.

The intervention was a success. The meeting was painfully heart-wrenching and emotional, but in the end, Ivan agreed to admit himself to a rehab center for thirty days, and he never touched alcohol again.

This event was a turning point in our marriage. Ivan saw me as a strong woman, and he often felt I could handle emotional situations better than he could. He would frequently challenge me about some of our household plans, but he always deferred to my judgment if the matter was emotional for him, the kids, or other family members. I also saw this newfound strength in myself and came to believe I could control most outcomes and overcome most difficult situations.

In 1991, I joined Ivan in the creation of our own company that handled employee benefits for corporations, including human resources and benefit administration. Within two years, we bought out the other two partners, and I led the outsourcing unit for the human resources team, among other duties. Our business was a huge success, and in 1999, Ivan became the CEO, and I became the president. Over the next three years, I managed to increase the profitability of the company by five times our original margin, and this impressed Ivan. He had initially expressed concern about my nonconventional business ideas, but the staff responded positively to them, and the success proved to be a direct result of my efforts and approach.

I was extremely happy during this time. I loved our company, I loved the insurance and human resources work we did for our customers, and I loved trying new ideas to motivate the staff. I felt my life was perfect. Ivan talked about selling our business and retiring, but I knew we were enjoying the benefits of our success, and I did not believe we would sell in the immediate future. The girls were doing well in college and business, we had two vacation homes—one in the Napa Wine Country and another near Yosemite—and we were active members of the board of the Fremont Chamber of Commerce. Ivan and I were happy in our marriage, and we enjoyed frequent outings with close friends and neighbors. Our life was full.

Unfortunately, our idyllic life was about to change.

On September 11, 2001, I was in Colorado on a business trip to pursue some business ventures. I was awakened by my friend, who informed me that the New York Twin Towers were being attacked. We watched in horror on our television as a plane slammed into the second Twin Tower, as well as the other horrific events that continued to unfold that day. My flight was canceled, as all flights that day were grounded, so I made the decision to board a train from Colorado back to the San Francisco Bay Area, where Ivan could pick me up.

I boarded the train around 4:00 p.m. and fell asleep around 10:00 p.m., but at 2:00 a.m. on September 12, our train collided with a freight train that was attempting to divert off the track onto a side area. The impact was devastating. The engine and several cars piled onto each other as the rest of the passenger cars zig-zagged across the rails. The momentum of the railcars behind our car pushed us a second time into the front of the train, and I was injured attempting to brace myself when this impact occurred. The collision occurred at the Salt Flats in Utah, and the area was pitch-black as I exited and ran from the front of the train. People from the small town in the area came out to the site and shuttled us to the auditorium of a local school. Our injuries were triaged there, and we were placed on buses to travel several hours to Reno, Nevada, where family members were expected to pick us up.

My injury was a compressed nerve in my neck, which caused the loss of movement of my left hand. My arm felt like it was broken. I was given a neck brace, a sling for my arm, a wrist brace, and heavy medication. Ivan met me as I exited the bus, and Alison was by his side. They were both stunned by my appearance, and as we traveled the four-hour drive home, I explained the chain of events following the train accident. I was still experiencing post-traumatic stress from the accident and was in a state of high anxiety on the winding road toward home.

A couple of days after we arrived home, Ivan handed me a document that needed my signature. It was our letter of intent to enter into an agreement to sell our business. I was flabbergasted. In the months preceding, we had prepared documents for potential buyers of our company, but we had not discussed the timing or any of the possible buyers. His timing for all of this was horrible. I loved my job. I loved our staff. And I did not want to sell our business. Ivan stated that because he would be turning sixty-five soon, he did not want to continue to work. He wanted to retire, and he felt I could continue my work with a new owner. This broke my heart. We had spent over ten years together building our company, and our business relationship was perfect. We complemented each other's style—Ivan had incredible business savvy, and I was extremely creative. I did not understand why he wanted to end all of that and give up our work together.

After a few more days passed, my sadness turned to anger, and I told Ivan that if he planned to retire, I would retire with him. I did not want to continue to work for the new owners. He accepted this, and we spent long nights talking about our future and where we wanted to live. My anger soon turned to excitement as we traveled with friends to Grants Pass, Oregon, and discovered an area nearby their home that we loved. We signed our final agreement to sell our company at the end of 2001, and in June 2002, we purchased a home on the Applegate River in

Southern Oregon. We sold our homes in Napa and Yosemite to focus on our retirement in Oregon.

Our new home had six and a half acres with a peaceful setting by the river. The view from our backyard was of a tree-lined hillside. The oversized rock fireplace, along with the large timber columns in the living room, made our home feel like a lodge. The back of the house had floor-to-ceiling windows, and the French doors off the living room opened to a covered porch that overlooked the river.

Our business agreement outlined our commitment to continue our services for the 2002 calendar year to transition our management. During that year, we were to introduce the new owner, reassure the customers, and maintain our block of business so that customers remained with the new owner. Our plan was to finalize our transition within the first quarter of 2003 and officially retire from our business at that time.

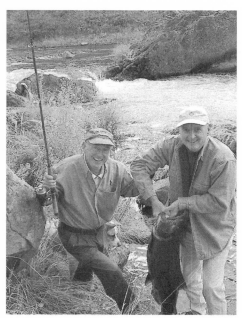

Ivan (on left) with his brother Charles on property

In October 2002, Ivan's oldest brother, Charles, visited us in Oregon. Charles and Ivan were close, and Ivan was proud to show off our new retirement home and the surrounding property. As they spent time together, they fished on the banks of our river and caught the largest fish in Ivan's fishing experience. This unexpected feat solidified Ivan's love for our new home, and he gloated about his success.

We were anxious to begin our retirement there, but during a trip to the home in December for the holidays that year, we received a call from our attorney, informing us about litigation initiated by the new owner: an attempt for a hostile takeover of the firm without payment. We were shocked and dismayed. The attempt appeared to have been planned. I later learned that the new owner was frustrated because I was not intending to remain with the firm after Ivan's retirement.

The first six months of 2003 were spent meeting with attorneys, dealing with court documents, planning the weddings of our daughters—Alison in June and Sara in August—and overseeing the sale of our home in Fremont in anticipation of our final move to Oregon.

I was angry over the litigation and wanted to fight to recover our ownership and penalize the new owner for his deceit. Ivan did not want to fight the action, and he continually tried to mediate the process. This upset me, as I felt that Ivan was giving up, and I didn't understand why he was retreating rather than fighting. This became a continual conflict between the two of us over the six-month period until a meeting one day with our attorney. While in his office, our attorney turned to me and said, "You need to stop fighting. Look at your husband. He's done with this."

I turned and stared at Ivan and saw for the first time a broken man who looked tired and sad. I realized then that he had wanted me to stop, but he needed our attorney to intervene. Feeling defeated and abandoned by both of them, I had a pit inside my stomach, and I felt like evil had just won over good. Despite these feelings, though, I knew I could no longer fight either. I needed to be done, too, so we began to discuss mediation.

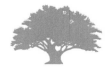

Chapter 2

Moving Day

The days, weeks, and months leading up to our July 25, 2003, move were stressful. I was feeling more and more apprehensive about our retirement plans because I had worked continuously since I was seventeen years old. Friends even joked that I was a workaholic. Work was my identity, and it provided an outlet for me to prove myself as a successful woman.

These doubts had added anxiety to the previous six months, which included preparations for the weddings of both daughters, the litigation to defend against the intended buyers of our business, and the sale of our home—which, by the way, we had been trying to sell in a newly downturned market. I was trying to create the perfect weddings for both girls without being consumed by the anger I felt over the litigation. I was in a constant emotional roller coaster, flipping back and forth from anger and grief to love and excitement. In the midst of it all, money seemed to be flying out the door.

Just prior to our move, Ivan felt ill and thought he might have a throat infection. We both downplayed how he was feeling, believing the stress from the first part of 2003 was at the root of his sore throat. We soon learned otherwise.

Three days prior to July 25, 2003, Ivan had a biopsy on his right lymph gland behind his ear. Although we had to admit that the apparent swollen gland could be an issue, we were so engrossed in the details of our final move that we convinced ourselves the results would not get in the way of our plans. With the impending move from California to Oregon, the start of our retirement years, the completion of Alison's wedding three weeks earlier, and the final planning stages of Sara's wedding that would follow in just a few weeks, our minds were filled with an overwhelming amount of details. There was no room for other worries, most especially Ivan's health.

It was a warm summer day. Ivan and I were caravanning in the two large rented moving trucks: he as the driver of one truck and me as the driver of the other following behind. I had our three-year-old cat, Pursy, in a carrier inside the cab floor. Our five-year-old dog, Ditto, sat on the seat next to me. The trucks were packed with the remaining belongings to be moved to our new home in Oregon. We had sold our home of the previous sixteen years in Fremont, California, and were excited to finally call Oregon home and enter this next new phase of life.

We had stopped about halfway into the trip for gas and coffee and were standing by the trucks sipping our coffee when Ivan reached over, pulled me close, wrapped his arms around me with a smothering hug, and told me he had received a call on his cell phone moments before we stopped…from the doctor. The biopsy, he had been told, was malignant. Cancer.

I pulled away from him in disbelief and immediately ran movie after movie in my mind, as if I were on some fast-moving train. I replayed the visits to the doctor, the mornings when Ivan complained of being tired, and the nausea he mentioned. As each memory flashed across my mind, I asked myself why I had not realized that he was seriously ill. I felt devastated, and I wanted to throw up. But even in that first moment of shock, I knew I could not show that emotion to him. I needed to be strong—for him. Unbeknownst to me, I had just been handed my new role—caregiver—and I'd accepted.

As we resumed our caravan, I called our close friends in Oregon, Jean and Vince, and cried as I told them about our devastating news. I could not hold back the tears. I was exhausted from the loading and packing process and had no reserves. I asked Vince to call Ivan. I knew Ivan would not reach out to anyone. Since Vince was his close friend, I hoped he would talk to Ivan and ask about how he was feeling. I knew Ivan was tough and didn't like to share his feelings with others, but because I felt devastated, I expected that Ivan must be hurting too. Maybe he would be willing to open up to his friend.

I was overwhelmed, wondering how just the two of us were going to unload the trucks in our current states of mind, but mostly I was disappointed in myself. Why had I not seen this coming and figured out how to manage it sooner? I felt guilty that I had been so self-absorbed in all the other events that I hadn't taken time to look at Ivan's physical appearance. I also felt alone—terribly alone—because I believed it was going to be up to me to *Take Care of Ivan*, to manage our move into our new home, and to find new doctors for Ivan as I continued to manage the remaining details of Sara's upcoming wedding.

Outwardly, I was able to cry openly in the truck without Ivan seeing me. Inwardly, I was mad at Ivan for getting sick and adding this additional work to my already overflowing plate. This news was a sucker punch to the gut, and I worried about how I was going to manage the onslaught of new challenges.

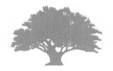

Chapter 3

The Wilting Violet

I was the youngest of four children, and my parents instilled in all of us deep-seated beliefs about strong work principles and the importance of family.

My dad had been a big band leader during the forties, and he continued to practice his trumpet every Sunday morning after breakfast. I recall fondly my early childhood when, sometimes after dinner, my dad would declare it was time to "parade" the neighborhood. We would scramble to grab pots, pans, spoons, or any other noisemakers we could find and line up behind him. He would start playing "When the Saints Go Marching In," and we would follow behind him with our marching-band steps, banging on our individual noisemakers. Neighbors would open their doors as we marched up their walkways, and we would march around their living rooms before exiting toward the next neighbor. People always found this activity funny, but they seemed to enjoy it. I especially loved this family bonding time. It was fun and often filled with laughter. Humor and music were a huge influence on how my family interacted.

My father was a high school dropout, but he became a self-made man who was extremely successful in real estate and insurance. His strong cultural influences included his middle-class,

German-regimented upbringing that he transferred to us. Dinner was always at 6:00 p.m.; the girls were responsible for the house-work, and the boys were responsible for the yardwork; chores were always performed on Saturday mornings before we could play with friends; and he needed to approve any departure from this routine.

My mom transferred her cultural upbringing to us as well. She was the only girl with two older brothers, and her family was extremely poor. Her father had been an alcoholic, and she would share stories of heartache and frustration about her childhood. Control was her escape and survival mechanism, and she prided herself on keeping an extremely clean house. She was also an excellent cook. We were expected to make our beds every morning and go to church every Sunday, as well as during special religious periods. She expected us to behave or she would apply stiff dis-cipline, usually with a wire hanger that she used like a switch. She frequently reminded us that she had four children under five within a seven-year period, and this required a strict regimen for most aspects of our upbringing.

Sunday night was always a formal dinnertime in our dining room, and my parents used this time as a teaching moment. My dad would instruct the boys about wine selections, table manners, or proper ordering for their dinner dates. My mom also used the weekly dinner as a chance for my sister and me to learn how to set a formal table, including the use of certain dinnerware and the correct manner to signal to a waiter/waitress that we were finished with our dish, simply by how our utensils were placed on the plate. We were even taught how to properly eat soup and cut our meat. If we accidentally placed our elbows on the table, my mom would sharply smack our arm with a spoon. Typically, at the end of every Sunday dinner, my dad would tell jokes and invite us all to join in. It was fun and lively, and I looked forward to this part of the meal.

I believed I had learned to be positive through my father's attitude. I had come to believe that positive people don't acknowledge depressing or negative things. I believed that if I gave negative thoughts any importance, they could become real. Thinking of them could make them happen. I believed that in order to conquer negative thoughts and prevent them from happening, I needed to be strong and work hard at positive thinking. In hindsight, my so-called positive attitude was probably my way of living in denial and avoidance.

As I grew up, my father called me a "wilting violet." He gave me this name because I cowered whenever I was placed in a situation where I needed to speak up and tell people what I was thinking. My whole body would shrink, shoulders slumped forward, and I would speak softly, if at all. Although I hated this title, I think my father used it to try to discourage me from having this reaction.

As I reflect on my father's reaction to my behavior, vivid memories snap into frame of dinner conversations, when he attempted to teach us simple math percentages. He would fire questions at each of us, asking us to answer a math problem. As he pointed to one of my siblings and asked, "What's five percent of a dollar?" they would fire back the answer. I hated this exercise. I did not like math, and the very nature of his approach intimidated me. I would freeze by the time he pointed to me for my question. I typically did not know the answer, and although he would stop and try to help me understand how to do simple math in my head, I could not hear him. I could see his lips moving, but I wasn't listening. I was busy talking in my head and telling myself I had failed.

As I got older, this wilting reaction diminished, but I remained apologetic, frequently saying "I'm sorry" for both little and big things. I did not want to disappoint people. I believed saying "I'm sorry" showed that I cared about others above myself. I did not feel worthy to stand up for myself. These feelings and beliefs would shape the way I interacted with people as an adult, including my husband Ivan.

I felt inadequate and inferior to my other siblings. My oldest brother was extremely athletic, and my older sister was a straight-A student. My other brother was charismatic and a mathematical wizard. I was none of those things. I loved sports, but I did not excel like my brother; I was a B student when I applied myself, but I felt I was not as smart as my sister; I was an introvert who felt uncomfortable in large social settings and could never be as gregarious as my other brother.

By the time the word "cancer" was declared that day, those childhood thoughts and beliefs about myself were deeply rooted. And in the weeks and months that followed, I believed that I needed to become strong enough and smart enough to come up with the answers to every question if I was going to succeed over this new adversary and manage this new role. Unfortunately, my self-doubt and sense of inadequacy would continue to influence my reactions.

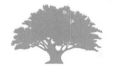

Chapter 4

All About Strength

Ivan was born and raised in Arkansas and was the middle child of seven brothers and sisters. He was raised with strong religious beliefs by his mother, who was Baptist. His family was extremely poor, and he told stories of being baptized in the river and sleeping in the same bed with his three other brothers.

When he was in high school, he shared a funny story about wearing his older brother's blue suede shoes. His brother had worked hard to earn enough money to buy the extravagant shoes, and when he saw Ivan wearing them, he chased him onto the school's football field and all the way home.

In a darker story, Ivan's mother told me of a time when Ivan and a few friends were caravanning to a high school social. Ivan's girlfriend was in the car in front of the car he was in. They

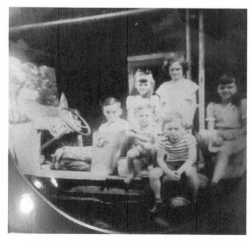

Ivan (front) and five of his siblings –
around 1946

traveled on dirt roads to the gathering. At the railroad crossing, which did not have crossing guards, her car was hit by an oncoming train, and everyone in that car was killed. Ivan's mother told me that it was the only time she saw Ivan weep openly and uncontrollably.

He adored his mother, but the struggles of the family were a strain. His father drank excessively and was abusive. His mother struggled to make ends meet for the family. Around the age of eighteen, he left home and headed west with hardly any money in his pocket. He found work in Southern California as a claims adjuster for an insurance company and spent most of his career in the insurance industry. Ivan had a strong desire to succeed in business and show his mother and siblings he could overcome adversity.

In 2000, Ivan's mother passed away. Years earlier, she had divorced his father, moved to Oklahoma, and become a full-time caregiver for an elderly woman. When the woman passed away, his mother received the woman's home as compensation for her service. This was the first time his mother had ever owned a home. She talked to Ivan frequently, as they maintained a close bond despite their physical distance from one another. We traveled to Oklahoma for her funeral, and Ivan was quiet and stoic until he walked up to the open casket. As he looked down at her, he wept.

Ivan had a dry sense of humor and was a highly intelligent man. He felt he could do better in life than his father, who had been less than responsible toward his family. Ivan was a proud man and rarely asked for help. He wanted to show others that a poor country boy from Arkansas could become a successful businessman with wealth. He was determined to make this happen.

In May 2003, when Ivan turned sixty-five, planning his retirement was a dream come true. The move to Oregon meant everything to him. He had succeeded in earning enough money to retire; he had found the perfect home on a river in Oregon, where he could spend his days fishing, golfing, or relaxing; and most of all, he had proven to his siblings that he was a success.

With the news that he had cancer, Ivan's inward retreat was profound. He didn't speak much about what he was thinking or feeling. How betrayed he must have felt. All that he had worked so hard to create was being challenged, and he would have to fight to keep it.

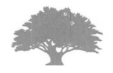

Chapter 5

What's in a Word

I have read and heard people make statements that I believed were overly dramatic, such as, "I couldn't believe it was happening to us," or "That situation changed our lives." But there I was—this *was* happening to us. I had always tried to avoid drama, as it typically brought attention to me. I also tried to avoid other people's drama. Since drama usually involved negative or sad situations, I avoided these whenever possible. But there we were, involved in our own drama, and those dramatic statements seemed very real and relevant to me.

The news didn't seem real. I may have said that I understood and accepted that health issues could hit us one day, but I never really believed they would. They happened to other people—people I heard about in social conversations—but not me. And since I'm a positive person, if this were true, I believed we could beat this with a lot of effort and intentional, positive thinking. So, from the moment I reached our home in Oregon, I scrambled to regain control of our lives.

Back around 1969, women who married were expected to stay home, raise children, and take care of the household. When I was seventeen, my father stated that he hoped I would be lucky enough to get married because I wasn't smart enough or strong enough to succeed in business. He wasn't trying to be mean; he was just struggling with his concerns about my future. He had witnessed my consistent cowering, my less-than-stellar performance in school academics, and my lack of passion for any specific profession. He was worried, and at that point, so was I. My brothers had enlisted in the navy, and my sister had received a scholarship for the University of San Francisco. My siblings had a plan, but I did not.

However, my father's statement burned an impression on the inside of my eyelids, and I started my business career determined to prove to my family (and myself) that I could, in fact, be successful. Based on my childhood, I believed hard work and focus were critical to my success. And as I progressed in business, job after job, promotion after promotion, this proved to be true. I taught myself to type, I taught myself to read new computer software systems, and I studied and learned the workings of the insurance industry. I explored positions that were above me and taught myself whatever I needed to learn to achieve that job. When other employees reported to me, I sat with them and learned every aspect of their job as if I needed to perform that job myself. I obviously didn't need to do that, but this practice helped me to understand many of the details within the various aspects of insurance and catapulted me into my own position. As I gained strength in knowledge and performance results through this type of diligence and effort, I believed I could control the outcome of my life.

Control was a large part of my belief system. I believed control was a critical element to successful outcomes. Control your outlook on life, and you control the outcome. But cancer? I was afraid of this disease. At the age of twenty-one, I saw cancer take my father's life. I had been unable to control that outcome. My father did not want people to feel sorry for him or make a big deal about his illness, and my mother respected him by reminding us not to speak of the illness with him.

I can still recall sitting at the kitchen table one night, having dinner with my parents, when my dad bolted up from his chair to race to the bathroom. The bathroom was just off the kitchen area, and as my mom and I sat motionless, not lifting our forks or saying a word, we listened to my father retching and heaving in the next room. I glanced at my mother, and she quietly mouthed, "Don't say a word when he comes back."

This was cancer to me: an unspoken illness that requires quiet strength and complete control. This is what I learned from my first encounter with this disease. My father struggled with cancer for over a year as he declined in weight and energy. My sister often visited from college, and my brother stopped by for coffee almost every morning. I was not a very good support person for my mother during my father's illness, though, because I was too caught up in my own issues.

I had married in 1970, and after two years of marriage, my husband had asked for a divorce. He informed me of his decision during Memorial Day Weekend of 1972, the same weekend we learned of my father's illness. Doctors had been treating my father's condition for what they believed was an ulcer, but my mother called me that Sunday night and informed me that they had diagnosed cancer, and my father was given a few months to live. I was devastated. My husband was leaving, and my father was dying.

Initially, I did not want my parents to know about my failed marriage. I felt they had their own problems, so I kept my situation a secret for several weeks until I could no longer hide my sorrow. Unbeknownst to me, my husband had been having an affair, and in the days following that unfortunate weekend, I learned more and more about his indiscretions from friends. I was devastated.

Over the period of sixteen months during my father's illness, I only remember a few poignant moments when the sadness about my father's condition overwhelmed me. However, I still never expected my father to die. I always believed he would win his fight against the disease. As the months passed, I finalized my divorce, remarried, moved into a new home, and started a new career in the insurance industry.

I married Jim in June 1973, but this marriage was an unfortunate rebound from the rejection of my first marriage. My father must have seen this because the night before the wedding he sat on the edge of my bed, saying he could help me by calling off the wedding. How did he know I was not in love with Jim? How did he see through my deception and the facade of a happy union? I didn't let him stop the marriage. I lied and told him I was in love, but after he left the room, I cried myself to sleep, fearful of my ability to maintain this lie. I wanted so much to be loved, and Jim loved me, so I was determined to try.

In March 1974, during the last days of my father's life, my mother, two brothers, sister, and I sat beside his hospital bed in a steady vigil. He was so frail and thin that the main artery along the side of his neck protruded dramatically. We watched this vein pulse as he remained heavily medicated. When my father passed his last breath, and the vein along the side of his neck no longer moved, the nurse asked us to step out of the room. As she came out and informed us he had passed, I ran to my mother to hug her, but she pushed me away angrily. My brothers and sister yelled at her to stop, and with that, she broke down crying as my oldest brother held her. I apparently went into shock. I don't remember anything that followed. It was hours later when I found myself at my parents' home, crying into my husband's shoulder. Jim had been at work in San Francisco, but when they called him and told him I was in shock, he left work, and within a couple of hours, he reached me.

My father had been the foundation of our family—the hard-working man with the humorous personality. People loved him, and he had many friends and business associates. He had instilled in all of us a strong sense of strength and pride toward achieving success, but then he was gone. How was it possible for him to lose this fight with cancer? Didn't the good and the strong always prevail? I was twenty-one years old and extremely naïve. It took me years before I realized that the answer to this question was no.

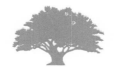

Chapter 6

Figuring It Out

That was 1974, but then it was 2003, almost thirty years later, and I was scared. I wanted to be that wilting violet again. I wanted to retreat and hide from cancer and all that came with it. Other friends and family members were also diagnosed during this same time, and it was simply too hard to understand that this was happening to me too.

Within the same month as Ivan's diagnosis, the husband of a friend was diagnosed with cancer and my stepfather was told he had lung cancer. The friend died quicker than expected after his diagnosis, and my stepfather's health began to decline drastically as well. I worried that our fate might follow theirs.

Ivan and I had only just begun the next phase of our life together—a time in life that many people dream of. Retirement represented leisure time to enjoy hobbies, sports, and time together. The word "cancer" instantly crushed all of that. I wasn't sure how I was going to fight this. And there was so much to learn about Ivan's cancer. *How was I going to learn what I needed to know and learn it fast?* The overwhelming burden of what lay ahead made me want to go inward. I curled up on the inside, wilting once more and struggling to stand up straight. I wanted to be that wilting violet all over again since I worried that I was not smart enough or strong enough to win this fight.

After first hearing the news in July and throughout the next few months, we traveled several times back and forth from Oregon to the UCSF Medical Center in San Francisco, California. Our doctor in California had referred us to an oncologist in Medford, Oregon, but he also suggested that we travel to San Francisco for further tests.

Our initial trip to San Francisco was heartbreaking because the doctor's office was full of patients, the clinic was sterile and unfriendly, and the tests took a toll on Ivan's strength. In Oregon, we had further tests, biopsies, doctors' visits, and assessment after assessment. We met with oncologists, radiologists, urologists, and all their interns in training. They all probed and scoped and pressed on Ivan.

I also searched the internet for information pertaining to his form of cancer and treatments. But despite it all, we were out of control. I knew it. Or at least I should say "not in control," and that seemed wrong somehow. There I was, not sure what to do next. I was a person who needed to stay busy by "doing something that needed to be done"—reading, learning, or taking action to resolve a matter. We were doing all we could, and yet negative results and reports continued. Doctors told us that surgery on the lymph nodes was unlikely, kidney issues could mean chemotherapy was not possible, and the location of the cancer could result in a widespread issue. So, I began to ask, "Why us? Why Ivan? Why me?" I worried over these questions and wondered if God had forsaken us.

I was a strong Catholic. I believed in God. But I began to ask myself, "Where is God now?" I had dutifully raised our children to believe in God and follow the practice of that faith. Ivan was also spiritual and believed in a higher power. He used to repeat a favorite line of his often: "God has a schedule, and He's on time." Yet, why was this happening to us, and why was it happening then?

Was this a punishment for not behaving in some way, or was there a schedule that would show others how good people are exalted?

My belief about putting others above myself became more pronounced. I was determined to show people and prove to myself what a good wife I was—a strong, capable wife. I believed I could conquer this illness by working hard and keeping positive thoughts. My husband and I had worked hard to achieve retirement. Cancer was trying to rob me of my right to be happy, and I was not going to let it win. Admittedly, I was angry. I had given up my working career for retirement—not for this. *This* was unfair. As angry as I felt for these unexpected and overwhelming circumstances, I also felt guilty for thinking those thoughts, but I kept it all to myself.

Friends and family began calling to find out about Ivan's test results and our general well-being. The easiest way to share the information seemed to be through a group email. This approach was helpful because it meant I did not have to interact with people directly. It allowed me to appear strong and in control. I feared that if I spoke with people, I would break down and cry. I was scared, but I needed to keep that to myself too.

I also needed to do everything I could to help Ivan through this. I told myself that what was happening wasn't about me. This was happening to him, and he needed my support. He needed to see that I could remain strong and steadfast in the face of cancer. Of course, that wasn't true. I needed support, too, only I could not and would not let others know. Weakness was my burden, helplessness my cross. I had struggled with these two beliefs most of my life and continued to believe that I needed to show up, strong and self-sufficient. So I decided I would do what I had learned to do since childhood: I would not show my feelings about cancer to anyone.

Once I decided to start the group emails, I told myself that it needed to be about the facts only. The importance was in the information I conveyed, noting the date and time of day for each transmission and the people who were participating in the distribution group. The following is the first of the series of email transmissions to the group.

> *8/20/2003   11:34 a.m.*
> *To: Health Watch Group (11 people in group)*
> *Subject: Ivan—Update*
> *From: Suzanne*
>
> *Hey Guys,*
> *   Good news. The tumor board confirmed that the tumor appears to be squamous cell and the treatment plan should be as originally proposed. [Radiation / Chemo and then surgery].*
> *   We're waiting for the Radiation Oncologist to call now to tell us if she can recommend a doctor in Medford, so Ivan can stay home during the 7-week radiation program. He's happy that we don't have to travel to SF and that he can recover in his own bed!*
> *   I'll keep you posted on any new developments. Thanks so much for your prayers and thoughts.*

Initially, the desire to avoid personal interaction and to not have to feel others' or my own sadness compelled me to write these emails. In the beginning, some people wrote back or called me to express their condolences, but eventually, Alison told people to reach out to her if they needed any additional information. Alison had told me of her decision to shield me from additional unwanted contact, and I was grateful.

I continued to write the email updates and found that they made me feel good because I was doing something productive and helpful, especially since I thought these emails would be read by Ivan after he overcame his illness. Writing them to chronicle his journey back to health gave me a greater purpose and made me feel strong. I needed this added benefit, so I could avoid being scared.

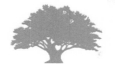

Chapter 7

Far, Far Away

Our daughter Alison is a loving, five-foot-three brunette who was twenty-six years old at the time of Ivan's diagnosis. She and her husband, Kye, had married in June 2003, the month before our move, and they were busy with new jobs and a new home in the Sacramento area. They lived about five hours from our home in Oregon. Although she was from my prior marriage to Jim, she was two years old when Ivan and I met, and he adored her. From the moment we found out about Ivan's health condition, she tried to support me and relieve me of some of the emotional pain.

Our other daughter, Sara, was born when Alison was six years old, and Alison immediately thought Sara was *her* baby. She became Sara's "other mother." Her caring, loving nature was evident even back then.

Sara was born on June 1, 1983, around a year and a half after Ivan and I married.

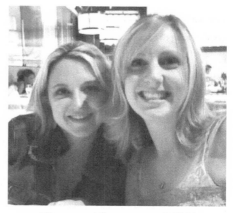

Alison and Sara around 2001

She is a five-foot-eight, blonde, extroverted, energetic woman who was twenty years old at the time of Ivan's cancer diagnosis. She and her husband, Kevin, married in August of that same year, the month following our move to Oregon, and they moved to San Diego. Sara was busy completing her college education, and Kevin was in the navy.

At the time of Sara's wedding in August, Ivan was already in so much pain from some of the tests that had been performed on his throat and glands that he was unable to attend Sara and Kevin's rehearsal dinner. Ivan was also beginning to experience a sharp and constant pain that radiated from his right side neck lymph gland to his temple, and this made movement difficult. Knowing that her dad was too ill to attend the rehearsal dinner was extremely emotional for Sara. She wanted to be strong and celebrate her impending marriage, but she broke into tears during her speech and presentation of a gift for Ivan and me. She read the book *The Giving Tree* and shared how much that book paralleled her life with us. She had painted a picture of a tree and framed it as a wedding gift to us.

There wasn't a dry eye in the restaurant. The entire group of people that had gathered to celebrate the engagement and wedding was all thinking of Ivan, who was back at the hotel, feeling ill. They looked at me with heartbroken eyes, and I tried to help them feel good about their participation in Sara's celebration. The focus needed to be on Sara. This was *her* night, and I wanted them to be happy for *her*, so she could be happy and not think about her father.

The day of the wedding, I needed to be with Sara early in the morning. Because I had to leave, a close friend came to our room, helped Ivan dress, and brought him to the wedding site. Ivan was in pain but managed to walk Sara down the aisle and attend the reception that followed. During Sara's father-daughter dance with Ivan, they played a prerecorded speech from Sara to her dad while the song "It's a Wonderful World" played. This was Ivan's favorite song. Alison openly wept, as did many of our close friends, when they heard the words Sara spoke to her father.

I walked to the other side of the reception area because I could not watch them dance together. This was heart-wrenching and poignant, and I knew I would not be able to stop if I let myself begin to cry. I was scared, sad, and in a state of disbelief about the seriousness of Ivan's condition, and I didn't want others to know this.

After the wedding, Ivan and I drove back to Oregon, where we would be alone and on our own. We lived far away from family and friends, and everyone was busy. Our daughters and their husbands (who coincidentally were brothers) were starting their new lives together. My stepfather had been diagnosed with lung cancer only months before Ivan, so my mom was busy attending to his needs. My brother and sister still worked, but because they lived near my mom in the Bay Area, they were supporting my mom, as well as managing their own families. And since no one, including me, thought Ivan was critically ill, it didn't seem necessary to direct their time and attention toward us. As Ivan and I attempted to manage his health situation on our own—and I attempted to downplay Ivan's condition—I didn't think we needed to impose on anyone else.

At the beginning of our initial doctor visits to San Francisco for test results, I began to shelter others from information that I thought was too negative for them to hear. I tried to give information that I believed was helpful, but what I failed to report to the entire Health Watch Group was that the California doctor had told me that Ivan had a 40 percent chance of survival. During that encounter, I was alone in the hospital waiting room.

The doctor came into the room, called me into the hallway of the treatment center, and as various people walked by, he told me about the biopsy results—the cancerous growth on the back of the tongue, the fact that the right side neck lymph node was enlarged, and that any future surgery would be precarious at best, due to a location near the nerve endings. Ivan was not with me when the doctor informed me of all this. He was resting quietly after his procedure.

I stepped outside the hospital building and wept openly, my face in my hands. I didn't care who saw me. I didn't know anyone there, and I needed to release my emotions and acknowledge my fear before returning to Ivan's room. This was one of the few times I allowed myself to let go and cry. But I decided not to tell everyone what I knew. After all, this would sound negative, and I needed everyone to be positive—especially me.

This need to stay positive would become a dance I would do time and time again: the dance of the smile, the dance of the strong, the dance of the good wife, the caring wife, the wife who was in control of the entire situation. I was none of these. I was crushed. My positive thinking was not enough to keep this bad news from us. I wasn't sure what to do next or how to move forward.

I had attended a program on positive thinking, intention, and the art of abundance back in 2002. Alison, Sara, and Ivan had also attended this program, so they knew I was a strong believer in the power of intention. I had seen several successful examples of this in others, as well as in our lives, so I tried to apply this knowledge and the required behavior. I needed to suppress the feeling of disappointment. Yet, I knew that emotion all too well.

As I replayed my earlier life events, I recalled feeling disappointment in myself when my parents shook their heads in disgust the night I told them I thought I was pregnant (and unmarried). I was almost eighteen and terribly in love, but watching my parents' reaction was heart-wrenching. I married Paul, my first love, just after high school graduation, but fortunately, the pregnancy test had been a false read.

I recalled feeling disappointment in myself when Paul announced he was leaving me for another woman, that he had never loved me and had only stayed with me until he finished college. I worked three jobs to put him through school, and I was madly in love and blinded by that love. Although his words cut through me like a knife, he said them to get me to stop pleading with him to stay.

I recalled feeling disappointment in myself when I was fired from a job after working hard to maintain the responsibilities I'd been given. I had accepted this new position at a different company despite my reservations about the manager. I was miserable because the manager treated me poorly. Clearly, I was so unhappy that my performance suffered, and I was ultimately let go. I had never been fired, so this outcome was a chink in my armor. I'd always tried to show others that I could succeed.

When I arrived home, my second husband, Jim, was happy that I had been fired and stated, "Good. Now maybe you will stay home and take care of our one-year-old." I hated him at that moment. Little did he know he was confirming my father's statement earlier in my life, that I was not smart enough or good enough for business. I filed for divorce from Jim as soon as I secured a new job in San Francisco.

Yes, I knew disappointment, and I cringed at the thought of failing in my war against cancer. I believed disappointment was the same as failure, and preventing failure meant everything to me. Ironically, I believed cancer was my war, not Ivan's. I felt this was my fight, not his, and it was important for me to win. Winning the war on cancer could redeem me from my past.

In my mind, Ivan was supposed to sleep and get well. I was supposed to fight the fight and cure him. How distorted this sounds today, but this was my truth at the time—the internal message I told myself. I was his caregiver. I needed to be more powerful than cancer, so I straightened my back and became determined to win.

After the initial tests had been conducted at UCSF, we talked to the California doctor about the diagnosis and the best place to start his treatment. We were informed that a new cancer center had just opened in Medford, Oregon (about forty-five minutes from our home). The physician in California told us we were "lucky" because of our proximity to this new center, and, in fact, he knew several doctors he could have us call to start treatment in Oregon.

I was happy to learn about the new center for more than one reason. First, we could stay in Oregon and manage the illness from the comfort of our own home, and second, the waiting room at UCSF in California had been devastating and depressing. That waiting room was full of people who clearly had serious illnesses, and some of them showed the obvious removal of facial sections or body parts. It was frightening. Also, our experience in California had made us feel like we were just a number in a long line of people who were waiting to see the doctor before they died. It was difficult to feel strong in that facility.

We decided to check out the new cancer center in Medford and were pleasantly surprised by the uplifting atmosphere and openly friendly staff. People who were visibly ill were not filling all the chairs in the room. In fact, the room was an enormous lobby that was decorated much like a hotel. People were reading, working on jigsaw puzzles, and engaged in pleasant conversations with cups of coffee in their hands. We were greeted at the door as we entered, and when they discovered we were there to view the center, they gave us a tour of the facility, helping us to understand how the various areas were designed. We were shown where the families could wait and even the special rooms for each patient, so they did not have to wait in the general area.

The new center was adjacent to one of the hospitals in town, Rogue Valley Hospital, and Ivan and I both felt immediately relieved by what we saw and the people we met. This environment made us feel hopeful that things might turn out okay. We began to think positively about the steps involved with the cancer treatment process, and we were confident that the efforts of physicians and staff would lead to a perfect outcome. All my thoughts of Ivan's chances of survival were covered up by this positive place.

8/27/2003   *8:36 p.m.*
To: Health Watch Group   *(17 people in group)*
Subject: Ivan—Update
From: Suzanne

We went to our first visit with the Radiation Oncologist and the session took approximately 4 hours. [they were very thorough]

    There is a lot to absorb right now—but I'll try to update you in a way that works best for each of you.

    For the people who do best with the simple information [just read this]:

    Radiation treatment should begin in about 10 days. We are being connected to a General Oncologist for the Chemo treatment, which will run at the same time. Radiation will be 5 days a week for 7 weeks. Next week we will be set up with a nutritionist, the Chemo doctor and the group who will "map" out the radiation plan. To map the plan out they will take a CT scan and another MRI and a computer will map out the exact placement of the rays based on the tumor sites, etc. This also takes a couple of weeks to complete in order to begin radiation. Recovery will be another 2-3 months following the radiation / chemo treatments.

    Now…if you prefer MORE details—I can tell you a little more [but don't feel bad if you prefer to stop here…it's ok].

    For those of you who want more information:

    First—I would suggest a great website: http:// orbit.unh.edu/cancer

    This site outlines everything from the beginning stages [treatment, tests, etc.] to surgery, nutrition and other points. It also has pictures in some of the pages—so be prepared. The doctor said that this is one of the most difficult treatments any cancer patient will have to undergo—because of the location of the tumors.

Ivan will have to have a tube placed in the stomach next week or the week after, where we will need to inject liquids/food during treatments. [His mouth will be too sore after a while to eat.] As treatment progresses he [or I] will have to inject him at least 8 times a day.

He will also have to have a tube in his neck area near his clavicle for the chemo treatment. The chemical is too strong to use the regular intravenous feeding method, as it would ruin the veins.

Ivan will not be able to speak once the treatments pick up the pace, as his mouth will be too sore—so only e-mail or letters will be his form of communicating as long as he's not too tired...which brings me to one of the last points. The radiation will make him tired and after the first few weeks this tiredness will increase and increase. The doctor said he will feel too tired to eat and food will taste like cardboard—but he has to eat as much as he can for as long as he can. He has already lost 6 pounds in the last 2 weeks because of his loss of appetite and the doctor said this is not ok during treatment. The body needs to replace the cells they are killing with the radiation and if he's losing weight—the body won't do what it needs to do to replace the cells.

The nutritionist will help us learn about foods we can try. He can't eat anything with acid [tomato, juices, etc.] He needs protein, even if we have to blender everything we can to get it down.

The radiation will cause him to permanently lose facial hair in the area around the treated areas—and Chemo may cause temporary loss of hearing. He won't be able to wear his dentures for the entire treatment and for a couple of months after. After that they will probably need to be refitted apparently.

A couple of months following the end of the treatment they will be able to check to see if the treatment was successful. It takes time for the body to process the dead cancer cells from the tumors and so we will have to wait before they will run further tests to learn the results. At that time, we will learn more about any decision for surgery.

On a final note—his prostate infection has not improved so I took him to urgent care yesterday and they are running another test to see if the type of infection should be treated with a different medication. They also put him on one medicine that caused a severe reaction and had us back in the urgent care room 3 hours later. He is on several drugs now for that issue and they indicated that it will take 7-9 weeks to recover. [just an added bonus for him to deal with right now].

Well—I think that's it…I apologize for the lengthy message. Let me know if there is anyone else that would like to be added to the 'health watch group'. It's so much easier for us this way but please feel free to call when you need to.

We love you guys and thanks for thinking of Ivan and keeping him in your prayers.

I felt strong writing this email because I had information about the treatment and his condition, and this felt empowering. I was careful to provide "just the facts, ma'am" because I didn't dare share my feelings of fear and anxiety. This might cause people to feel sorry for me and Ivan, and I worried that such a reaction would weaken my fight against this very strong adversary. If they felt sorry for me, then I might begin to do the same. Besides, no matter what, I needed to stay positive.

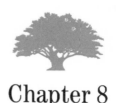

Chapter 8

It Starts

A nd so, it started: the many months of email transmissions
that would begin to unfold the health of my husband and
the chronicling of our journey into *The Twilight Zone.* For that
is what this was: scary, monstrous stuff.

The Twilight Zone was a television series back in the sixties.
It was a collection of frightful science fiction tales that included
Martians, monsters, and unexplained events about people's greatest fears. This was my greatest fear: to lose the man I loved. It
seemed as if I was watching a TV episode about fear itself, only it
was my fear—fear of being alone out in the country in a new and
different state, fear of what was expected of me in my role as the
caregiver, and fear of the many unknowns within the medical field.

In the beginning, there was a lot of information about what
the process might look like and the possible treatment plans.
To keep fear at bay, I told the story of what was happening in a
very matter-of-fact style. After all, I needed to be strong and stay
positive. These were just steps—a process—and I somehow felt
detached from it all. But there was a new unknown we were
soon to discover—the fact that the treatment plan could change
drastically with just the slightest change in the patient. Before
his illness, Ivan weighed 150 pounds. Even before the start of his

treatment, he began to lose weight. His weight became a marker for all of us: of how well he was or wasn't doing.

9/02/2003   *6:58 p.m.*
To: Health Watch Group   (25 people in group)
Subject: Ivan—Update
From: Suzanne

There is still a lot happening—so I'll try to update you as best I can [and hopefully I won't leave anything out]. Several people have also been added to the 'health watch group' and we are happy to include you!

We met with the Medical Oncologist and she gave us a slew of new pills for Ivan to take now and during treatment. Most are vitamins or pills that will help the production of cells. She also said that there is usually more than one tumor with this kind of cancer, so they are going to run a CT scan on Ivan's head, neck, chest, and lower track [in light of the recent problems]. They will also do a bone scan. These tests will specially look for other tumors. The tests are scheduled for 2 on Wednesday, 2 on Thursday and 2 on Friday.

Ivan sees the Urologist on Thursday for that problem. Friday, they place the Porta-Cath in the clavicle area for the Chemo injections [as I mentioned before].

A week from today [next Tuesday] Ivan will go into the hospital and they will insert the stomach tube in place. He will have to stay overnight for them to monitor any possible rejections, etc.

The doctor has told Ivan he has to stop smoking A WEEK BEFORE treatment begins—but, odd as it may sound to most of you; this is his biggest problem right now. Stress makes him smoke more and the thought of stopping has him really fearful and anxious.

The Radiation Oncologist / Chemo doctors think we will be able to start treatment within 10 days, so we are gearing up as best we can. Blood tests, supplies, you name it—we're trying to prepare for what we may need.

Since Chemo wipes out your system—we were told to be prepared for the "unexpected"—such as infections or other medical problems. People who have had family members with this type of cancer have offered their information too, which has been really helpful. [Electric comforter —because he will be really cold as a result of the radiation; walkie-talkies—so Ivan can beep me when he needs something while he is in bed, since he won't be able to talk; cold-water swabs by his bed for his mouth—since he will lose his saliva glands, etc.]

As soon as we hear the results from the various tests as to the extent of the cancer and if it has traveled elsewhere in his body—I will let you know. Other than that—Ivan is starting to get nervous about the future treatments and he has become more quiet and inward.

It's amazing the number of people who have stepped up to send their prayers and best wishes. He and I are overwhelmed by our friends and family!

Thank you for being there for us and let me know if you have any questions.

Since the process began, I'd felt personally responsible for Ivan's life, driving him to the appointments, picking up prescriptions, and learning how to properly administer the various foods and medicines. This was not a problem. After all, I saw this as my role in his illness. I was retired, so I told myself I should be able to do what was necessary to support him. I tried to minimize everything else I needed to worry about, including our new home, the lawsuit regarding the closing of our business, the dog, the cat, adjusting to our new surroundings, and finding my way to the various appointments. I reminded myself that Ivan needed to be strong to fight the disease, and I needed to follow the doctors' instructions as the caregiver.

As the intensity of the treatment increased, I felt the need to increase my knowledge, as well as my strength. Ivan's pattern was to manage the challenges inwardly, and my reaction was to learn as much as I could, so I would be smart enough to fight this cunning enemy. Being defined as the caregiver carried a tremendous weight; it was a heavy burden that I tried to minimize and accept without question. I believed that everything I did had to be done correctly or Ivan would suffer the consequences. That, in fact, turned out to be the truth. We would soon learn that any action of the caregiver has an impact on the patient, whether good or bad. Ultimately, both of us would come to share the anxiety about the illness *and* the process.

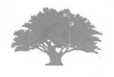

Chapter 9

Lost

During one of the tests in California, Ivan developed a separate health issue due to a problem with his catheter. Because of this new and painful issue, we were told to schedule an appointment with a urologist in Medford. Although we were also in the process of setting up his cancer treatment plan, this situation needed to be addressed right away to relieve his pain.

After living in the area for only a couple of months, our travel around the city had been limited, due to the need to stay at home and allow Ivan to rest. An appointment for an MRI had been scheduled to map the radiation treatment around the neck glands, and this was a critical step in beginning the course of treatment for the cancer.

On September 4, 2003, an appointment with the urologist had been scheduled, followed by an appointment for the MRI. Both time slots had been difficult to schedule, so we were grateful that they could happen on the same day since it took almost an hour to get into town for these appointments. Unfortunately, because of my unfamiliarly with the area, I had trouble finding the urologist's office. I had to rely on maps of the Medford area, and I was unclear about the exact route to take to their office. The time we lost in trying to find the doctor's office created a problem for the subsequent MRI appointment.

When we arrived at the MRI office, fifteen minutes past our appointment time, they would not accept us and required us to reschedule the appointment for the following week. Since the MRI was required before radiation treatment could begin, this was a huge setback. I cried for hours once we returned home, feeling that I had let Ivan down and that I had shirked my caregiver responsibilities, somehow not taking them seriously enough.

I felt extremely guilty, and it took several days before I could shake this feeling. Tremendous guilt had always accompanied simple mistakes, and although I had made a simple mistake by not mapping out the location of the urologist's office ahead of time, it was clear to me that the impact on Ivan would be huge. A delay in treatment would allow the cancer to continue to grow.

I also felt that when I exhaled, twenty other family and friends breathed out with me. I continuously received inquiries about Ivan's health since they were anxious to stay abreast of his daily progress. Because family and friends were not able to visit us, I believed they were placing their hopes and wishes on me for a successful outcome. They constantly asked me to *Take Care of Ivan* and to keep them updated about his progress.

They were riding this emotional roller coaster with us, which made me feel that I was somehow accountable to them, as well as to Ivan. This added accountability created an additional burden because I felt that I was being *watched* by the Health Watch Group and that I needed to perform at the highest level so they would be proud of me. I needed to be the perfect caregiver and wife that everyone was expecting me to be, and yet I did not feel like the perfect caregiver. I was battling my fear of the possible loss of my husband and our failure to beat this disease. I was battling my own demons, and self-doubt continued to grow. The seed of the added pressure of meeting the expectations of others was a burden that would also continue to grow over the next few months.

9/09/2003   *7:01 p.m.*
To: Health Watch Group   *(33 people in group)*
Subject: Ivan—Update
From: Suzanne

Today, as you know, Ivan had surgery to install the stomach tube. The procedure went extremely well and Ivan will stay in the hospital overnight. The dietitian set up a meal plan for the tube feedings [which the doctor has instructed us to begin right away]. We will have to inject 9 cans of Ensure® a day through the stomach tube, in addition to his regular meals, about every 2-3 hours. I learned how to do the injections and it went very smoothly. Although the site of the tube is painful right now, Ivan is doing well and we are looking forward to having him back in his own bed tomorrow.

The test that we took on Monday apparently had a problem and they have requested that he retake the test Thursday. Other than that—we wait for the doctor meeting on Friday to learn of the results and the next step.

I'll keep you posted as we learn more information.

Learning how to administer Ensure® into Ivan's stomach tube was empowering and gave me a deeper sense of purpose and direction toward his recovery. Although some people responded to my emails, letting me know they were sending their prayers and waiting with bated breath for my next communication, I focused on what was in front of me. I busied myself with household chores, Ivan's injections, and his daily care. By keeping busy, I was able to find peace and quiet and solitude from people who wanted more information about Ivan's progress. This was avoidance, I realized, but this form of solitude helped me to remain in denial about the severity of the situation we were facing.

I also had another new challenge to manage. Ivan's mood had changed, and he was becoming more and more impatient. The feeding protocols consisted of using a syringe to check for any residual from the former feeding. If there was residual, it meant the previous fluid had not been processed yet, so adding more would make Ivan throw up, due to the overload of fluid in his stomach. If there was no residual, I could insert the syringe of Ensure®, which had been filled to a set amount marked on the side of the syringe, and dispense it gradually into the stomach tube. This process started out slowly as I attempted to feed him two ounces at a time, repeating the feedings to achieve eight ounces per day. The entire process was painless for Ivan, but he was irritated and frustrated by the slow process that had to be repeated every three hours.

The feeding process was stressful to me, too, because his stomach was not processing the liquid in the amount of time expected, so I was unable to get in more than four to six ounces a day. Yet, because Ivan needed to maintain his weight as part of the battle against cancer, he was supposed to get a minimum of eight ounces a day. Each time I checked for residual and found that I could not add more liquid, I felt frustrated too.

Not wanting to share our challenges and my frustrations with everyone, as people replied to my emails or sent me inquiries, I tried to respond with upbeat news, but this was difficult. Due to the chores I needed to tend to around our property, as well as Ivan's daily care, I usually managed the emails late in the evening. I hated to tell them a lot about what was really happening because I didn't want them to know how much I was truly struggling with our situation and my own emotions. This created an extra burden for me to carry—another self-imposed cross for me to bear.

9/18/2003   1:14 p.m.
To: Health Watch Group   (39 people in group)
Subject: Ivan—Update
From: Suzanne

This is a hard e-mail to write, since the news is not good.

The results of the re-take test for the kidneys indicate that his kidney function has, to quote the doctor "drastically deteriorated". She said she can no longer consider Chemo therapy and she has consulted with the Radiation Oncologist to increase his dosage of radiation in the later part of his treatment.

We have set up an appointment with a Primary Care doctor for Monday, and hopefully this physician will direct us to what we need to do next to turn the situation around.

Ivan is disappointed—to say the least—and he can't talk about the results right now. He's angry and frustrated that his health is not what he thinks it should be, and so the mood in the house today is a little somber.

We are not giving up—just taking a break to regroup in order to take on this new issue. I need to get on the Internet and look up kidney failure so I am prepared for the new 'twist' that we will experience together, if that's where we will be going.

Thank you for your prayers and support though. I know I always say 'thank you'—but I'm sure you don't realize how much your e-mail, thoughts and prayers are helping right now. Without this contact and support, I think this home would feel empty and lonely—so thank you...truly.

This day was yet another turning point for Ivan and me. The punch in the stomach we both felt when the oncologist told us about the kidney results was devastating. And another factor entered the mix—Ivan's darkening mood. We had always been close and respectful toward each other, but he began to lash out at me, and I was struggling to understand why. I took the angry comments personally, and his curt, angry tone resulted in me retreating almost daily to the back room for a good cry. I believed that during this time in our lives, the two of us needed to lock arms and stay close. Yet, I felt he was pushing me away, treating me as if I were saying or doing everything wrong.

I realize now that it was his only way of venting his frustration and anger toward his ill health and his body, which was not cooperating. (He later commented that he felt his body was letting him down.) But to be pushed away by the very person I loved and wanted to protect was painful. When Ivan lashed out at me, it felt as if he was disappointed in me and did not want me around. I tried to strengthen and solidify our love and show him

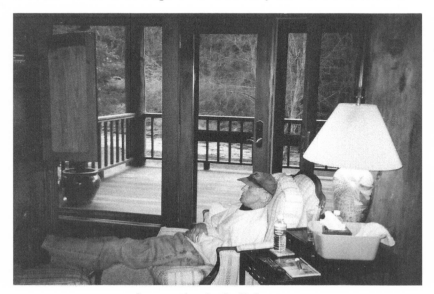

Ivan resting in the living room

what a good wife I was, and I felt he was rejecting me. It was hard to understand what he was thinking and feeling. Since he did not openly share his thoughts and feelings, I was left to make up things in my mind, which always seemed to shine a negative light on my actions. I felt that I was failing, that I was a big disappointment incapable of managing this situation, so the tears flowed often and privately in the back room.

During one of the visits by his sister, Shelby, who came to help around the house, she witnessed his anger and my retreat to the back room. She followed me to the back and hugged me as I sobbed. She spoke of the emotional reaction and rationalization for Ivan's anger toward his illness and his body's betrayal. Shelby reminded me about Ivan's long history of working toward retirement, only to be facing a life-threatening condition instead of the days of relaxation he'd anticipated. Her words stuck with me. It would take several weeks before I would shift emotionally from the hurt I was feeling and accept the fact that his anger, while directed at me, was *not about me*.

10/01/2003   *6:54 a.m.*
To: Health Watch Group   *(39 people in group)*
Subject: Ivan—Update
From: Suzanne

Good morning. I want to update you on what has been going on but I want to be sure I put a positive spin on what I say. We need positive energy right now.

Ivan has been feeling nauseated and has been vomiting the past few days. Monday was his first radiation treatment but as fate would have it the machine broke down before he could complete his treatment and it ended up a long day for him [5 hours] instead of 30 minutes. But the good news is the treatment has begun.

Because he was feeling so poorly by Tuesday morning—I took him to the General Oncologist and they found his blood pressure was 217 over 107. He also now weighs 128. To help him feel better [so he can eat and keep the Ensure® in him] they gave him a medicine pack through the porta-cath and it helped. They gave him new pills to take and they sent him home to rest and let the medicine work, so we did not have a radiation treatment on Tuesday.

They are not sure why he is vomiting now, since that is not a symptom related to the cancer he has, but we see the Internal Medicine doctor Thursday and hopefully he will be able to identify the problem.

For those of you who may call, you will find his voice has changed again as he is a little hoarse. The doctor said this is due to the cancer in the tongue nerve.

His sister and brother-in-law came to visit for a few days and that was great.

Other than that—I would like to ask each of you to say a prayer for Ivan that the new medicine will help him feel better, that he can accept the Ensure®—all cans, and that his weight begins to increase. This is where we need the energy most! And we know such powerful friends, I know this will happen.

I'll try to let you know more information, if we learn anything new by the end of the week.

Close friends and family called often to ask about Ivan and me. Sometimes I let them talk to Ivan, but most of the time he did not wish to speak, due to the pain he was experiencing. I sent this particular email early in the morning because we had a couple of errands and appointments that would take up most of the day.

One of the errands was my driver's test and a new Oregon driver's license. I took my photo for the license, and that document, dated October 1, would be a constant reminder in the months and years to follow of what transpired on that day in 2003. Little did we realize that Ivan's body had been trying to tell us something in those preceding days; little did we know how our world was about to be turned upside down.

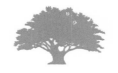

Chapter 10

October Moon

The week of September 19, 2003, our daughter Alison and her husband, Kye, had come up from California to Oregon to help around the house and see Ivan. Since our move in July, we had spent most of our days at doctors' offices, so having the kids come to visit for the first time was a welcomed relief.

Ivan took Kye down to the river in our backyard to spend a short time fishing. On the way back from the river's edge, apparently, Ivan slipped on the rocks and fell. He complained that his left side hurt under his rib cage, but he became angry with me when I asked about the injury or suggested that we get it checked out. He insisted it was nothing, and so nothing was said again.

Around 6:00 p.m. on October 1, Ivan began to complain that he did not feel well. He had been sitting in his chair watching television but said he was going to lay down in bed. Moments later, he cried out to me to, "Come quick!" and when I entered the bedroom, he was rolling back and forth on the bed, telling me he felt funny and that his side was in intense pain. I had him sit up so I could check his blood pressure with our monitor, but the situation was quickly deteriorating. While seated, his eyes rolled back. He fell to the ground and became unresponsive, despite me shaking his shoulders and calling his name. My heart raced. I immediately dialed 911. My fingers shook, and it was difficult to hit the correct numbers. As I continued to yell Ivan's name, hoping he would respond, I informed the operator about what was happening and gave her our home address.

She spoke in a slow, calming voice; however, this situation was anything but calm. I needed to be with Ivan and try to wake him, but she kept asking me for information that I thought was useless and unimportant at the time. I needed to use the phone to open the automatic gate and allow the ambulance access to our property, and she would not let me hang up. I felt anger and fear at the same time. Here was my husband, lying on the floor, and this woman on the other end of the line wanted to ask me silly questions about what had happened. With shaking hands, I hung up on her, tossed the phone onto the floor, and raced to the front door. I left it open for the paramedics I hoped would come soon, dialed the access code to open the property gate, and ran back to Ivan's side.

Once the paramedics arrived, in what seemed to be long, excruciating hours (but was only about ten to fifteen minutes), they immediately stabilized Ivan. They could not gain a pulse, although he was awake and responding to their instructions. He casually looked over at me from time to time and shook his head disapprovingly, with disdain, because I had called for the paramedics. He was embarrassed. He wasn't the type of person who would ask for help, and I had caused him to look weak in someone else's eyes. He was truly mad, but I knew I had done the right thing.

He was taken by the ambulance to Rogue Valley Hospital, about forty-five minutes into town. As I followed, alone in my own car, I desperately tried to reach each of my daughters or my brother and sister, but no one was home. It was difficult to drive and select a phone number as I attempted to reach someone—anyone. I finally reached our friends Pat and Sharon, who lived in California, and explained the situation. My voice shook as I spoke, and I held back my tears. I needed them to find my girls and let them know what was happening. I spoke in brief sentences as I told them Ivan had been taken to emergency. By the time I pulled into the hospital parking lot, they agreed to contact our daughters, and we hung up the phone. I ran into the hospital to find out where they had taken Ivan, and nurses pointed to one of the back rooms in the emergency room area.

I spent the next five hours in the emergency room with Ivan while they assessed him, drew blood, and tried to determine why he was in pain. Throughout those five hours, Ivan complained and asked me to do something. Nurses and technicians entered and left the room to perform their tests, but most of the time, we were alone in the room while Ivan moaned and rolled from side to side, trying to get comfortable. He complained that he was cold, his left side was in pain, and he was extremely uncomfortable and could not get any relief.

Finally his oncologist—whom we had only met a couple of times—appeared at the doorway of the room and asked me to step into the hallway. She informed me that Ivan had lost a considerable amount of blood: three pints to be exact. He was obviously bleeding internally, but they had no idea where. She said the situation was grave and that I should call my family. He was later moved to intensive care, given a blood transfusion, and stabilized. ICU began running tests, but the doctor informed me again that she felt the outlook was extremely poor.

This was a turning point, I would later realize, in our fight against the cancer. As we battled to save Ivan's life from this new health issue that had presented itself, the fight against cancer stopped.

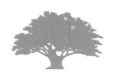

Chapter 11

Hard Day's Night

As I sat with Ivan in his ICU room, my mind kept flashing back to the visual of Ivan's eyes rolling into the back of his head, the paramedics trying to find a pulse, the moaning and twisting as he tried to get comfortable on the hospital gurney, and the look on the doctor's face as she told me to call my family because "things did not look good." I was petrified that I could be left alone with no one by my side.

When I returned around 1:30 a.m. the next morning to our large, empty house in the country, I wrote an email to the Health Watch Group. In a strange way, the emails had become my connection with people, and at that moment, I desperately needed to feel a connection. My hands shook as I typed the email, and I had difficulty controlling my physical reaction to the mental pictures that continued to play in my mind. I would start to cry, straighten up, continue to type the email, and start to cry again. *Alone*—this possibility danced in my head, and I kept trying to dismiss it. I felt weak and helpless.

> *10/02/2003   1:53 a.m.*
> *To: Health Watch Group   (42 people in group)*
> *Subject:Ivan—Update*
> *From: Suzanne*

My hardest e-mail yet.

Tonight emergency took Ivan to the hospital. His health changed around 6:00 p.m. and so I called 911.

They are keeping him there while they try to improve his condition and run further tests.

Please think positive—regardless of where the mind goes. We need everyone to focus on Ivan's powerful style and picture him being stubborn and determined with the situation. Ok?

I'm mindful that I've asked a lot of all of you—to ride the emotional roller coaster through this ordeal. So thank you for being there for us.

I will let you know how his health progresses when I can.

I felt lost and alone. The solitude of the empty house and my emotional exhaustion from what had transpired added to these feelings. My email said nothing about the specifics of the episode that had taken place at our home, including the doctor's urging that I notify my family. I was wrapped up in fear and denial that I could lose Ivan. I had never before considered that Ivan might die. The harsh reality of the 911 event made me realize this was a very real possibility, and I felt helpless. I thought about the possibility of managing the household and our finances without him, of tending to the six and a half acres on my own, and the reality of the distance from all our friends and family. I felt sorry for myself as I experienced an overwhelming feeling of being alone. I thought about how we had created this situation through our decisions to move to this area and my portrayal of being a person who didn't need to depend on anyone for assistance.

It was almost 2:00 a.m. by the time I finished my email, and my heart pounded rapidly as I prepared for bed. I lay in bed, staring at the ceiling, as tears seeped out of the corners of my eyes and onto the pillow. I tried to tell myself that he was going to be alright, that I needed to continue to think positively. But each time I glanced over at where Ivan had slept just hours before, I wept openly. I did not sleep at all that night.

10/04/2003   *5:17 a.m.*
To: Health Watch Group (43 people in group)
Subject: Ivan—Update
From: Suzanne

As some of you know, Ivan's condition improved Friday—upgraded from critical to serious. However, last evening they identified that he is bleeding into his spleen, which they now found was the life-threatening cause for the 911 event.

As of this morning, they have also found the need to increase his oxygen—as his lungs appear to be filling up with fluid.

Later this morning the blood tests will tell us if he is continuing to bleed. If so, we have elected surgery—despite the fact it will be high-risk for Ivan. Surgery could occur today—we're not sure—due to the recent change in his lung situation, this may create a problem or if the spleen has stopped bleeding—and the need for surgery is eliminated.

I know Sara gave you our cell phone numbers— and it's been great having people check in with us when they need to know the status. When we step out to the parking lot for various breaks—we are trying to return calls or update people.

The navy has flown Kevin in to be with us so Alison, Kye, Sara and Kevin are here with Ivan and I. The Leonards are also here, running errands for us and helping where they can.

*Your prayers are important—so please don't feel
that you're not here with us too. You are.*

*Things are changing quickly from day-to-day,
hour-to-hour and we will do our best to keep you
posted.*

Once Pat and Sharon told Alison and Sara about their father's
condition, they called me immediately, and we arranged their travel
to Oregon. Sara and Kevin flew in from San Diego, and Alison
and Kye drove up from Sacramento. The four of them arrived the
following day. It was good to have our daughters close to us, to
have them see their dad and watch the process in the ICU that
became our world over the subsequent weeks.

As a parent, as well as a spouse, I felt an intense responsibility
to stay strong for our daughters, to help them remain calm and not
fall victim to grief or fear. Having the girls close meant I needed to
be "on," which was as tiring as the forty-five-minute drive back and
forth to the hospital. I wanted so much to tell them how afraid I
was, but I knew I wouldn't. I couldn't. I needed to keep my own fear
at bay so I could be strong for them. I think they knew I wouldn't
open up. They didn't ask—I didn't tell. This became the unspoken
message: they needed to be positive too—in the same way I had
participated in my own mother's handling of my father's illness.

Our friends Pat and Sharon had also driven up from the San
Francisco Bay Area. They and our daughters and sons-in-law
laughed and connected as they sat in the waiting room outside the
ICU. It was clear that they were enjoying each other's company.
Yet, the atmosphere struck me as odd—like a funeral reception
following the services, where people gather, talk, joke, and recon-
nect. It was hard for me to listen to their laughter, but I didn't let
them know. As much as I might have tried to join in their conversations, I couldn't, fearing that at any moment the doctor would
appear and announce Ivan's death.

As I sat there, waiting for what might happen next, I thought about what I wanted for our girls. These were our daughters, and I wanted them to be happy—not fear the worst. I feared the worst, but I kept it to myself. I continued to think about how I would manage the six and a half acres, our finances, and the girls' reactions to his death—alone. My self-imposed prison of positivity required that I keep my internal hell to myself.

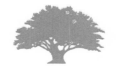

Chapter 12

The Lonely Road

The first night after the girls arrived in Oregon, they talked me into leaving the hospital and returning home to sleep. Our plan was to return to the ICU the next morning. At 4:00 a.m. on October 5, the loud ringing of the house phone broke the night's silence. The sound startled me out of a deep sleep, and my heart jumped as I quickly reached for the receiver. It was the intensive care nurse. She told me that Ivan's doctor wanted me to know he had taken a turn for the worse, and they were increasing his oxygen to help the situation. I hung up and immediately began to dress for the hospital.

The sound of the house phone ringing also woke the girls and their husbands, who were all staying with me at the house. The girls came into my room and saw that I was hastily getting dressed. They became concerned and asked if everything was okay. I reassured them that the nurse had called to give me an update—to let me know that Ivan just required more oxygen. I told them that I wanted to get to the hospital earlier than planned since I couldn't sleep. They seemed relieved by my tone and words and said they would go back to sleep and drive to the hospital later in the morning. I moved quickly toward the car, started the engine, and pulled out of our long driveway onto the two-lane road.

As on each morning since Ivan's hospitalization, the drive down the country road was dark, winding, and lonely—very lonely. The oncoming headlights of one or two cars were the only lights that periodically lit the road. Along parts of the road, the overhead night sky was hidden by the overhead branches of large oaks and dense pine trees. Porch lights from neighboring houses were scattered along the hillside and down long driveways set back from the road. Mostly, the landscape was stretches of dark open pastures and tree-lined curves.

Driving back and forth each day, my mind focused on the surrounding bushes that flanked the roadside. I had been told gruesome stories of deer that darted out from behind the bordering shrubbery and caused unexpected accidents, which made this daily trek stressful. The darkness was heavy, adding to how I felt each morning. I was exhausted. When I drove to the hospital in the early morning, I thought about what I needed to ask each physician who would check Ivan that day. As I drove home

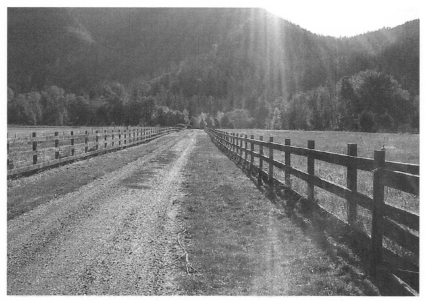

Long driveway towards our home

late at night, I reviewed the events of that day and thought about how depressing it was to watch my husband endure the pain and discomfort of the hospital bed.

I felt responsible for learning all I could about Ivan's condition, so I made sure I was in his hospital room during doctor rounds. The rounds were held between 6:00 and 7:00 a.m. each morning and again around 6:00 to 7:00 p.m. at night. I also made sure I was in the room during the nurses' change of shift. I learned, the hard way, that there were many times when the nurses were unable to transfer all the pertinent patient information, which led to the issuance of duplicate meds or missed meds. The nurses' shift change was usually over by 8:00 p.m. To ensure that I did not miss any of these crucial times, I needed to leave the house every morning around 5:00 a.m., and I typically returned home around 10:00 p.m. each night.

Ivan usually told the doctors and nurses to talk to me because I was the one handling everything regarding his care. He was tired and disappointed in his body, so he abrogated his role to me. This added to the pressure I felt to make sure I made the right decision at the right time…every time. I willingly accepted this role though. Being his eyes, ears, and voice gave me a clear sense of purpose. I was his ambassador, his advocate, his *savior*.

10/06/2003   *7:20 a.m.*
To: Health Watch Group *(43 people in group)*
Subject: Ivan—Update
From: Suzanne

I will make it brief as I have to drive to the hospital to be sure to see the doctors when they do their rounds.
First, you are an amazing group. Ivan has GREATLY improved yesterday and they have upgraded

his condition back to serious. When he caught pneumonia the doctors were not encouraged and not hopeful—but your prayers and ours showed otherwise.

Today I find out if his spleen has stopped bleeding and what the next step is. Each day we "take on" another organ in this chain of issues, but the results remain positive. He is sitting up in bed, working on his breathing and is less and less sedated. He has stopped being angry about being where he is and in fact last night was the first time I felt he was truly 'Ivan' again.

I will try to write tonight to let you know how today went—but I believe things have turned a corner finally and we will start to receive nothing but good news.

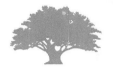

Chapter 13

Juggling

Following the 911 call and during the early days in ICU, Ivan's condition became precarious. As they struggled to locate the cause of the bleeding, he caught pneumonia from the increase in IV fluids. They also found possible blood clots near his heart that caused them concern, and they wanted to surgically remove them, if possible. But they could not perform surgery until they located and stabilized the bleeding. His kidney was struggling to manage the loss of blood, and he was quickly reaching the level of kidney failure.

There were as many as eight different doctors assigned to Ivan and ten different medications. Each physician was dealing with specific major medical issues, and each was asking me for my decision regarding how to triage the situation since there was no one doctor managing Ivan's entire case. This felt incredibly heavy, the burden of needing to make medical choices and decisions on matters I did not understand. I was not a heart doctor, nor a kidney doctor, nor a surgeon, nor a pulmonary physician. I knew nothing about stents, oximeters, bilirubin counts, or creatinine levels. And yet, each physician met with me and reviewed their approach and treatment. I was a caregiver, not a managing physician, but I was expected to be both. There was no other physician or person placed in the role of managing Ivan's complete medical situation, so they looked to me. They expected me to listen to the information and provide them direction.

For instance, the pulmonologist advised me that the excess level of fluids was causing a negative impact on Ivan's lungs and asked that I agree with a reduction of his fluids, so he could document the medical file for any future interactions from other medical staff. However, as the cardiologist evaluated Ivan's situation and determined what was needed, he wanted to make sure the heart was receiving plenty of fluids. This scared me: two conflicting opinions—two opposing approaches. One mistake—one decision in the wrong direction—could cost Ivan his health or his life. I was stoic as they spoke to me and I made decisions. I was fearful after they left the room, praying that I had done the right thing and made the right choice. This was another ball to juggle, and there were an overwhelming number of medical balls in the air as we managed Ivan's lungs, heart, kidneys, urinary tract, spleen, and, of course, cancer.

10/07/2003   *9:30 p.m.*
To: Health Watch Group   *(43 people in group)*
Subject: Ivan—Update
From: Suzanne

I'm never sure if I'm writing too much or not enough so please accept my apologies if I write too often.

Ivan's stats are all good right now.

The blood count is better so they believe the spleen may have encapsulated itself and it may heal on its own. They will watch this for a few more days before we even have to consider surgery—and this may not be an issue at all.

The kidney numbers are going back down, so the specialist is happy and they are continuing to monitor that matter.

The pneumonia is better and Ivan is at level 5 oxygen—from being at the maximum—so this is definitely better.

The doctors said he will be a few more days in ICU and then we'll see where he goes from there.

He needs to get up now and start to move around— but he has been too tired for this.

He was a little depressed yesterday—but today his spirits seem better.

He has a General Oncologist, a kidney doctor, a lung doctor, a pulmonary doctor and a surgeon all checking him out each day. Not to mention the many lab tests and nurse interactions necessary for the good of his health. We just love the medical staff here.

Sara, Kevin, Kye and Alison have gone home now and will resume their regular schedule. Ditto, our dog stays in the car during the day and she and I have become good friends with the lawn section in the parking lot during my breaks.

Have I told you how grateful I am for all the prayers? This is truly a miracle story when you know all that he had to conquer.

Take care and I'll update you if things change or when he gets out of ICU.

On the morning of October 8, the surgeon approached me and indicated that they believed Ivan had blood clots near or around his heart. He suggested that we perform a procedure to remove the blood clots by inserting a line through the vein in his right thigh. They would guide the line through the veins, locate any clots near the heart, and clear them. He believed the procedure would be quick and easy for Ivan and that it would relieve one of Ivan's medical issues. I agreed, and the surgery was scheduled for that afternoon. Unfortunately, this decision turned out to be regrettable.

The surgery to clear the clots had several consequences. One, they were unable to travel through the veins as they had hoped, due to the structure of Ivan's veins. The veins were twisted and blocked any proper passage of the line. Two, the dye they inserted to view the veins was a substance that was difficult to process by the kidney, the same kidney that was already in distress. Three, some clots were released by the line that entered the veins, but this was not a good thing, as these clots traveled to the toes and stopped there. They later found that these small clots caused gangrene in the toes, and Ivan's toes began to slowly die from lack of oxygen.

I felt the decision, decision, had been deplorable. This decision caused the kidney to be in extreme distress, and it could possibly shut down. This decision caused Ivan's blood pressure to rise, placing a strain on the area that was mending the spleen. This decision caused irreparable damage to some of Ivan's toes, which were in jeopardy of being removed. I was devastated and in agony. Although the physician had made the recommendation, I felt my approval had caused my husband more pain and physical distress. I had failed, just as I had in the emergency room when I did not tell the physician about Ivan's complaint of pain on his left side—the same side as his spleen. I later realized that if I had said something, they might have checked that area and identified the source of the bleeding earlier. As a result, guilt became my permanent companion, along with my sense of inadequacy.

Ivan's body was in distress, and there were new issues added to our already full plate. How could I tell people I had made such a poor decision that could have taken his life—the very life I was supposed to take care of and guard? How could I tell my children that I had been so stupid? They relied on me to care for their father and be his caregiver and advocate.

The kidney doctor was furious when she found out about the surgical procedure I had authorized, and she pulled me into the hospital hallway and yelled at me. She stopped when I broke down crying and told her I needed help since no one appeared to be overseeing his overall health. She'd had no idea that I was being asked to make medical decisions by physicians who were focused on their own specialty, not on Ivan. She'd had no idea that I already felt enormously guilty over the outcome of that procedure.

As I sobbed and told her no one was helping me or overseeing Ivan's health, she softened and said she realized I was in the middle of the various doctors. She felt horrible about her reaction and said so. She would become a friend and ally over the months that followed, checking in on Ivan and me frequently and asking if she could help me with any of the medical issues.

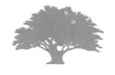

Chapter 14

Radiology

After being in ICU for ten days, Ivan's condition continued to improve, although the issue of his toes would never be resolved. Normally, gangrene is a significant medical condition, but with all the other health issues we were managing, this issue seemed inconsequential.

Prior to Ivan being admitted to ICU, he had begun his first treatment in radiology. His treatments had been scheduled for two times a week for about four months. Ivan spent two weeks in ICU, during which time he was unable to continue his treatment. The radiologist met with me outside ICU and informed me that once a patient starts radiation, it should not be stopped until the treatment is complete. He stated that if it is stopped, the cancer is stimulated instead of diminished. This information was frightening.

Treatments could not begin again until Ivan was transferred from ICU to the oncology ward. Because the radiation treatment was interrupted for two weeks, we feared what the doctor had told me—that his cancer had been stimulated—but we wouldn't know if this had occurred until the end of the full treatment.

Alison was being contacted by various friends and family who did not want to bother us. She informed me that people wanted to know about me, as well as Ivan. She asked me to send an email that shared what I was going through. This gave me permission to open up and let people know some of my own pain with cancer, but I struggled, not wanting to share too much. I wanted people to know that the situation was sad but not insurmountable. It was hard for me to focus on my own fears since I'd tried so hard in my life to appear positive and strong. I could not admit to my true emotions of loneliness, heartbreak, and even guilt. I had never before allowed myself to be vulnerable in front of others in this way and realized I still could not allow myself to do it, even then.

10/10/2003   8:23 p.m.
To: Health Watch Group   (44 people in group)
Subject: Ivan—Update
From: Suzanne

Ivan has been transferred from ICU to the Oncology ward! Once we finish up with a few minor issues [relatively speaking] we can go home. Maybe Tues of Weds [Can you believe it?]

It's a different kind of hard for us right now – not the worry and fear that it was before though, so I'm sure we'll get through this too. I'm usually tired in the evening from the long day at the hospital and when I get home it's hard to want to talk or write anymore. Hope some of you understand this is why I haven't written sooner or returned some calls. A little quiet time and a good cry usually help to make it easier to get up the next day and do it again. If you haven't experienced this kind of situation before—then you are blessed. To see someone you love in so much pain and daily difficulties is heart wrenching and takes its toll on us—but I'm keeping focused on him coming home and returning to the schedule we had set up for the treatments.

By the way, the treatments have resumed, even with Ivan in the hospital bed. The Oncologist did not want to wait and so they have been wheeling him into the radiation room in the bed and helping him to undergo the treatment.

I am grateful for the miracle of saving his life and now I ask that he be allowed to continue with as little pain and discomfort as possible.

I will write when I have more news. Take care.

I was exhausted with the routine, which was difficult to admit. After all, Ivan was the person who was going through Hell—not me. I was supposed to be grateful for my health and do whatever I needed to do to help him. But the process was taking its toll on me, and it was beginning to show.

I felt cancer was to blame for all that was happening, and it seemed to be winning. I began to gain weight, due to the late-night fast food and the poor food choices I made in the hospital cafeteria. The dark circles under my eyes were pronounced from the accumulated lack of sleep. My eyes were bloodshot and worn from my late-night cries. I woke up around 5:00 a.m. each day, fed Ditto, dressed, packed Ditto and her daily supplies into the car, and drove into town to the hospital. I got there in time to listen to all the reports and nurses' updates each morning and sometimes helped them with information about Ivan's care. Every four hours, I walked down to the car and took Ditto for a walk so she could relieve herself.

Ditto was an eighty-pound female, part Akita and part German Sheppard mix. She was five years old, and we had raised her since she was four weeks. She had been Ivan's shadow since she was a puppy. She was more than just a dog; she was a dedicated companion that was almost human-like. Ditto was sensitive, smart, and seemed to understand anything people said or did.

After we found out that Ivan was ill, Ditto's interaction with Ivan changed. She knew there was something wrong in the house—Ivan had changed. She no longer wanted to sit near him, leaning against his legs as she had always done. When he called for her to come to him, she would cower and immediately lay on the floor, careful not to make eye contact with Ivan. This was a sharp difference from how she had acted prior to his illness. She began to follow me around and stared at Ivan, as if she were afraid of him. Ivan was heartbroken by this display, but fortunately, the opposite reaction occurred with our cat, Purcy. Purcy would not leave Ivan's side. If he removed her from his lap or bedside, she would immediately jump back up, rubbing closely to his face and neck. Ivan had not been enamored with the cat, but her stubborn desire to be with him softened his view of her.

When we first moved into our new home, the six and a half acres were not fenced in for pets. The pasture had a cross fence, but there was no other mesh or fencing that would prevent Ditto from wandering out of the area. Ditto would not leave or run away when Ivan or I were in the yard. She always stayed by our side and was extremely mindful of our every move. Purcy remained in the house, happy to move from room to room or lay on a windowsill, staring at the birds outside busily gathering twigs or food. Unlike Ditto, she was content to be left alone.

My days in the hospital were typically seventeen to eighteen hours long, so it was impossible to leave Ditto in the house while I was gone. She wouldn't let me leave without her anyway. She loved to ride in the car and sat in the front passenger seat, her back straight against the seat. She did not stand up and hang

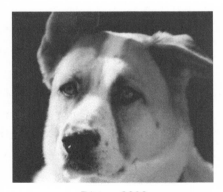

Ditto – 2003

78

out the window, as most dogs preferred. She did not like the window down or the wind blowing on her face. She continually sat in the seat and looked out the window as we drove. People often pointed at her and laughed because she sat in the seat, as if she were a person.

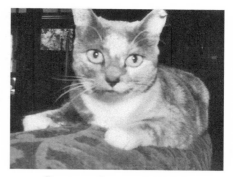

Purcy on the back of Ivan's favorite chair – 2004

I hated to leave Ditto in the car while I was in Ivan's hospital room, but I felt I had no choice. I could not find it in my heart to leave her with a pet boarding service. I did not know how long she would need to be there, but more importantly, she was my constant companion and I needed her. I believe she needed me too. She knew Ivan was ill, and although she cowered around him, she stayed close to my legs when we were together. She acted as if I were her safe haven.

In late November, the oncologist informed me that I could bring Ditto into Ivan's room. Ivan had been in the hospital for almost two months, and this suggestion sounded like it would be great for Ditto and for Ivan. Although other parts of the hospital did not allow animals, the oncology ward was different. They allowed dogs as part of the healing process and patient comfort. I was excited to reunite Ditto and Ivan. It proved to be a disaster, however. Ditto could not settle down. This otherwise calm and easygoing dog was nervous and frantic as she sniffed around the room. She raced from corner to corner and would not go near Ivan, regardless of how firmly he commanded her to do so.

Her anxious behavior continued for more than an hour. Although I hoped she would relax and lay down next to my feet, this did not happen either, so I returned her to the car. I believed that not only the stress of Ivan's illness was painful for her, but the strange smells and frightening, unfamiliar hospital room added to her discomfort. I never attempted a hospital visit with her again.

I visited Ditto at the car three times a day to take her out and walk her, so she could relieve herself and eat and drink something. While she was in the car, she slept. After a fifteen-minute walk with Ditto around the hospital grounds, I returned to Ivan's room and sat beside him. I accompanied him to any radiation treatments, x-rays, or scans that had been ordered the day before. I took notes regarding lab results and transferred the information to a spreadsheet when I returned home, tracking his progress myself.

On the drive home from the hospital around 10:00 p.m., I usually stopped at Kentucky Fried Chicken and ate my dinner as I drove along the country road. When I got home, I let Ditto out to run around, listened to voice messages, and managed my emails.

At this point, I was still managing the end of the lawsuit with our former business, so I also responded to any emails from the attorney. I typically collapsed into bed around midnight, but I was not able to sleep soundly. With the day's events still racing around in my head, I usually lay awake, planning the next step I needed to do to help Ivan return home.

Some nights, Ivan would plead with me to stay with him. He did not like being alone at the hospital, and I felt horrible telling him I couldn't stay. The fact was I did not *want* to stay. I longed for relief, at times feeling that the weight of the situation was more than I could bear. The drive home and my time at the house, however lonely and brief, were a break from the pressure and gloom of the hospital and Ivan's condition. Although I felt this was selfish, I had to admit to myself that I was exhausted and needed time away. Of course, this added to my guilt and sense of inadequacy for not being what Ivan needed me to be. I did not feel I was the "good wife" he thought I was. At times, I chastised myself, thinking that other wives would have stayed, but I couldn't. I continued to not feel good about myself.

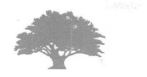

Chapter 15

A Nightmare

10/15/2003   7:04 a.m.
To: Health Watch Group (45 people in group)
Subject: Ivan—Update
From: Suzanne

I'm in a hurry this morning to drive to the hospital—but I wanted to request all of your prayers toward this new situation with Ivan.

I believe I mentioned he is still bleeding internally—and if I didn't, I'm sorry. Each day is something new. Sometimes good and sometimes not so good. If this were a novel—I would complain about the overkill on the hospital drama—but the surreal continues for now.

Yesterday Ivan apparently had a reaction to a medicine that caused his vital signs to drop drastically. The nurses worked on him and he was stable by the afternoon. However, they still don't know the cause of the bleeding and even if it's simple, they can't keep moving forward on their hunt for the problem until they get through certain steps.

So—please pray that Ivan's situation remains stable

That they are able to clear his system without further complications

That they are able to perform the two procedures today regarding a scope in his stomach and intestinal track

And that they can perform another CT scan to check the lungs and spleen.

Once these steps are accomplished—the doctors feel they will have a better idea what is going on—but this is the order.

There are so many twists, I can't begin to write them all, but I guess you realize Ivan will not be released this week as we had thought.

But as I write, I ask you to think positive again, as you all once did before. I believe it was your prayers

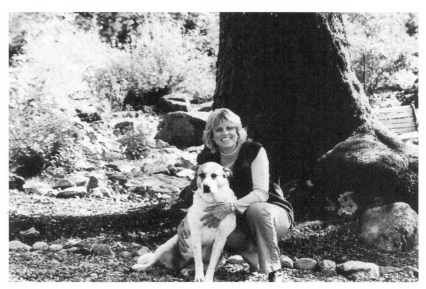

Ditto and me – Fall 2004

that saved his life before so I believe the joint energy works. Please help us again.

I will write again when I can—but no news is good news in that we ARE STILL FIGHTING to wheel him toward the front door of the hospital.

PS—He is at Rogue Valley Medical Center—for some of you who asked under separate email.

Thank you, as always, for your thoughts and prayers. We are eternally grateful for the people in our lives.

Ivan was heavily sedated, as he continued to be in a lot of pain from the tumor around the lymph nodes at his neck. It was putting pressure on the nerves in the area. He was not processing the Ensure® liquid either. The oncologist explained that in ICU they focused on stabilizing vital signs, not the intestinal tract. Although the medications they administered caused constipation, they expected this condition to be managed once the individual was released to another ward.

In Ivan's case, once he was transferred to the oncology ward, they began treatment for his intestinal tract. However, his system was not responding to the regular course of laxatives to clear his system. This began to alarm the doctors. They worried that the cancer had spread to his intestinal tract and that bleeding might be occurring in this area since blood loss had shown up again in the tests.

Ivan had to be watched because the pain medicine made him somewhat delirious, and he continually tried to remove the tubes from his nose, neck, and arms. At times, he would open his eyes and get angry with the person (the nurses or me), preventing him from removing the tubes. He had developed horrific bedsores on his lower back that had become open wounds the size of quarters. They required special ointment and treatment to prevent infection. This treatment was painful for him and difficult for me to administer. As his issues mounted, I became even more focused on the process rather than what I was feeling, which allowed me to manage the multitude of treatments and the care he needed.

The doctors decided to issue another dose of a laxative since the first dose had not worked. This became a nightmare once the medicine took effect. Alone in the hospital room, I began working with Ivan's body, as I tried to keep the bed and Ivan clear from the diarrhea that ensued. Heavily sedated, Ivan was neither aware nor able to help. The staff was shorthanded, and because this situation became unusually time-consuming, I was given pans and linens to capture the body fluids.

The process started early in the morning and continued well into the night and the following day. At one point, one of the nurses felt bad that I was managing the situation alone, and she helped me collect the fluids for about thirty minutes, but then she had to return to her regular duties. Alone again, I continued to collect, dispose of, and clean up the area on my own. The flow was constant, and my efforts seemed futile. But, although I felt helpless and overwhelmed, I had to keep at it so Ivan wouldn't suffer unnecessarily. There was no time to feel sorry for myself.

At this point, Ivan's bedsores were so pronounced around his anal area that we were unable to attach a fecal collection bag, which would have normally been used to handle the elimination process. He was losing a lot of fluid, and the doctor was extremely apologetic about having administered the extra dosage of laxative. They realized, too late, that his system was slower than normal, and that they simply had not waited long enough for the initial laxative to take effect.

On the second day, a business associate surprised me and stopped by the hospital room. She was an employee of a customer where I had been the VP of human resources a couple of years earlier. She lived in the area, heard that Ivan and I were in the local hospital, and decided to stop by for a social visit—just to drop in and say hi. She had no idea about the magnitude of our situation and the current state of affairs I was managing.

I heard a woman whisper, "Hello?" from the doorway, and I stepped out from behind the curtain that was drawn around Ivan's bed. He was completely exposed, and I held rags in my glove-covered hands. I was surprised when I saw her standing in the doorway, and I immediately asked her to please wait outside the doorway.

Since I could not allow her into the room, one of the nurses saw her standing in the doorway and took over for me. I took the unexpected guest to the family break room so we could talk. I was exhausted, miserable, and lonely, but I tried to sound strong and share Ivan's current health situation with her. Her presence caught me off guard, and it was apparent that she was caught off guard too. I could see from her expression that she'd had no idea about the severity of Ivan's illness. She was not a close friend; she was not part of the Health Watch Group. She was simply a person who thought she was doing a good deed by visiting someone she knew in the hospital.

I was not someone who shared my emotions freely, and yet, I found myself dumping all of my burdens onto this unsuspecting woman. I sobbed on her shoulder. I am sure it was a connection she had not expected, but I could not stop myself. In her embrace, my tears flowed. I would later reflect on the look of fear in her eyes as I told her about our situation.

Looking back now, I find this event both funny and depressing. Poor thing, she was a true deer in the headlights, but lucky me: I was finally able to release my pent-up emotions, even if it was to a person I hardly knew. The fact is I somehow felt it was safe to show my emotions to her since this poor woman was neither a close friend nor family. I didn't have a certain image I needed to maintain; I didn't have to pretend to be strong or capable; I could be myself and show my fear, sadness, and frustration about the current situation through my tears.

After this brief visit, I returned to the nightmare, where nothing had changed. I once again put on the latex gloves and took my place by Ivan's bed, relieving the nurse who had stepped in to help. Ivan's oncologist stopped by to check on the situation, and she asked a couple of nurses to help me. However, the first nurse insisted that she try to place the fecal bag on Ivan again, despite his obvious bedsores, and this attempt ended badly. As she attempted to attach the bag, her action was immediately halted by Ivan, who wheeled around in bed and grabbed her arm in anger. She froze as he stared at her. Although he was extremely medicated, he surprised all of us with his forceful action. He fell back onto his stomach without saying a word, and she retreated from the room.

What transpired with Ivan's body over those couple of days will forever be embedded in my mind. I don't remember or consider the situation disgusting or sickening in any way. I remember the situation as heartbreaking. Being unable to stop the flow of his bodily fluid or to keep his bed and body clear—this was truly an unsettling and dire circumstance. I felt sorry for Ivan on several levels—that another turn in the road had dealt him a bad circumstance, that his body was not cooperating with his desire to return home, and that he was void of any respectful, personal privacy in this situation, a key value to this strong-willed man. When this episode finally came to an end, I was emotionally and physically exhausted.

Once again, I felt responsible for his embarrassment, but I did not share what had taken place during those two days with anyone. The nurses knew. The doctors knew. But friends and family would never know. Being sensitive to Ivan's pride, this was not something I could ever share with anyone. It was another unfortunate moment for Ivan and another failure of mine.

I felt I had failed to direct the doctors away from their decision to administer the extra dose, and as a result, Ivan lost his privacy and dignity in front of the nurses and me. This was overwhelming to me since I was already carrying the burden of the previous medical decision that almost cost him his life. The misery, the embarrassment, and the guilt were difficult emotions to swallow, and I felt that I could hardly breathe from their weight. I was more fragile than ever, but I could not tell anyone. Once again, this was my burden to bear, no matter what.

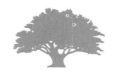

Chapter 16

Fight or Flight

10/17/2003   10:53 a.m.
To: Health Watch Group   (45 people in group)
Subject: Ivan—Update
From: Alison

Hello everyone,

It's Alison…today I am sending the email update for Mom…

Since she asked me to write this update, I thought I would take a moment to give you an update on her too! Mom is so thankful and comments on how supportive all of you are being for her and dad right now…but I am asking that we pray for her as well… she is really exhausted both mentally and physically. As you know she has been going to the hospital for 2 weeks. She leaves at 6:30 to get there by 7:00 a.m. and then usually gets home by 10:00 p.m. She doesn't want to leave dad's side. These past 5 days have been really tough for her and a true test of her strength. Many nurses are commenting on how amazing she is [which we all know].

On a positive note—grandma, Kye and I are here with her and she is really happy. We are keeping the house warm for her to come home to, visiting her at the hospital, making her favorite dishes (actually grandma is doing that...yummy) and doing some chores/errands around the house for her.

Now for the update on dad: I have always admired him and I do even more these days. He is a true FIGHTER. We are still waiting for more news from the doctors as they plan to do a CT scan today. Mom called a few minutes ago and said his vital signs are up today and that his coloring is looking better, so that is good news. However, his weight is still dropping and he currently weighs 116 .

We promise to keep you posted when we have any news. I like to keep thinking positive in that "no news is good news". As I mentioned above, mom is exhausted, so emails might be from myself or Sara. But please keep calls, emails, positive thoughts and prayers coming. We love you all and are so blessed to have the passionate, caring, loving friends and family that we have! We will write soon.

Having my family come to help was amazing. I was extremely grateful for their presence and their help. It felt wonderful to see the house lights on as I returned from the hospital late at night and drove up the long, dark driveway. It was a relief to see people waiting to greet me at the back door, to feel the warmth of the house and sense the smells of savory cooking. I was used to a dark, cold, and empty house when I returned each night from the hospital. This was a welcomed change that made me feel truly loved and not alone.

My mother had lost her husband of eleven years to cancer just the month before, so I knew she was grieving. Yet, she came up from Northern California to take care of me. She put her own emotions aside to care for me.

My mom was worried for me and felt compelled to be by my side, despite her own emotional pain. Just as she had always done in her role as a wife and mother, she stepped in and made sure I had food in the refrigerator, clean sheets on the bed, and a hot meal when I got home from the hospital at night. She cared for my basic needs. She had never worked in business but was a housewife and an incredible cook.

Ivan and my mom adored each other, and she was heartbroken when she saw his physical appearance in the hospital. The man she had laughed with, golfed with, and kidded around with was in tremendous pain, and this pulled at her heart.

Alison and Kye worked around the property, taking care of the yard and Ditto and helping Mom during the day. Alison also supported me emotionally in the morning before I left for the hospital and again at night when I returned. From the beginning, she had stepped in to have family and friends communicate with her so I could focus on Ivan's health. Each call required her to relive the pain she was experiencing and the pain cancer was causing, but she took on the responsibility anyway. This was Alison's style—to be a caring, emotional person who loved and worried about people.

Alison has always been a person who loves to hug people, but her hugs became even stronger with me. She would wrap her arms around me, squeeze tightly, and hold on. My heart broke whenever I looked into her eyes and saw her pain in reaction to my pain. I wanted to be strong in front of her, but her hugs were counteractive and disarming. As she hugged me, I felt safe and gave in to the tears that I had tried to hold back.

Although I was trying hard to maintain control, I didn't mind this brief release. I accepted it. Alison had the ability to disarm me, and I was grateful for that. The moment she held me, I melted, and the wall that kept my smile-mask on crumbled. I felt her love, which was overwhelming. I could not stay strong and emotionless. As hard as I might try not to, I always cried. Even today, when something is wrong, Alison's hug will reveal the true emotions behind my smile.

While my family was there, Ditto stayed at the house instead of traveling with me to the hospital since there was someone there to be with her, but they had to distract her until I drove out of sight each day. After I pulled out of the long driveway and onto the road, Mom would let her outside. She told me that each time I left, Ditto would race to the front and stand there, staring down the long driveway with her ears perked. She would hold that pose for several minutes, waiting and hoping to see my car, but eventually, she would give up and return to the back door to be let inside. No matter what time I arrived home, Ditto jumped up and raced to the back door, her tail wagging wildly and her body shifting from leg to leg, ready to run to me once the door opened.

10/19/2003   *9:31 p.m.*
To: Health Watch Group   *(46 people in group)*
Subject: Ivan—Update
From: Alison

Hello everyone,

It's Alison again…with the latest update.

Mom is doing better; still really exhausted and has her good days and bad days, but we keep reminding her that it's okay to cry. Grandma has made all of her favorite foods, which is good and she is really happy! And I am here giving her lots of hugs (she needs those right now) and Kye has gone back home to work.

I got to see dad today for the first time in 2 weeks. I must admit he looks different, but he is still the sharp Ivan we all know and love. Today, he was very concerned about making sure the nurse did not give him too much pain medicine so he could watch the niner game.

The CT scan showed that there is no cancer in his lungs which is great news and that the spleen is still enlarged but the doctors say it's nothing to be concerned about.

Dad is still in a lot of pain, which is really hard for mom to watch and for all of us to hear. He is definitely more alert in the morning and by the afternoon he is exhausted from the pain. This is what makes her cry because there is nothing that she can do to help. He is currently eating at 50% and they are trying to get him back up to 100% to put some weight on him.

We hope all of you are doing well! Thanks again for the calls and emails. We really appreciate them! I will write more soon. Hopefully we will have more information tomorrow.

Alison began to drive back and forth each weekend. She would drive up from Sacramento on a Friday and drive back on a Sunday, a six-hour drive each way. Her presence made me feel loved, and it was a relief to have someone in the house with me. The emotions that were roaring inside of me were becoming complex, so having one of my daughters by my side helped to quiet the voices in my head. I felt close to her, and she seemed to understand how forlorn I felt. I was able to share some of my feelings and fears, and although I realized I was placing an extra burden on her, the conversations helped to ease my sadness.

It was important to hug her too. I could tell she was getting more and more heartbroken about Ivan's circumstances, and she expressed her worry that Ivan might not survive this illness. I wanted to hold her in my arms, like when she was a young child, and tell her everything would be alright. I longed to give her encouraging news from the physicians, so I could ease some of her pain too. But she was a grown woman, and it was evident to me that the realities of the situation had not escaped her. She could see Ivan's deteriorating physical appearance. She could see the stress in my eyes.

Because it was hard not to cry in front of her, I felt guilty. Each time I cried or shared distressing news about one of Ivan's conditions, I felt heartbroken that I could not conceal my fears and allow her to remain positive and happy, as she had been before the illness. She had become my friend, my confidant, and my companion in this journey, but she was my daughter first and foremost, and I felt selfish for sharing this emotional roller coaster with her.

We did not talk about her own distress and emotional conflict, and yet I know she was also conflicted—wanting to cry but needing to be strong for me, wanting to share her fear of losing Ivan but being careful instead not to say anything negative. I didn't know how to manage such emotions with my child. I wanted to keep her close, yet distance her from the reality of this downward spiral. The very thought that my daughter was experiencing this horrific situation devastated me.

The visual that best explains my life's emotional path since the first day we learned about Ivan's illness is a descending line graph. Although I would get excited each time there was a high, I did not realize that the new high was not as high as the last one. And when we had a low, I did not notice that the new low was lower than the previous one. I believe the nurses knew it, and the doctors must have seen it, but it is only now, as I reflect back on our journey, that I can see it too.

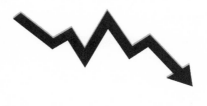

Each day at the hospital, I administered the liquid food every three hours through Ivan's stomach tube. I verified that the nurses were administering the correct medicine and providing it on time. In fact, on one occasion, a nurse came in to administer a particular medicine for Ivan, but thankfully, when I asked and she informed me about that particular medicine, I was able to stop the injection. This medicine had given Ivan a deadly reaction previously, and the nurse had not realized or paid close attention to what had been noted in his chart.

Whenever I was away from the hospital, I worried about Ivan's well-being and the potential mistakes of medical and nursing staff. After I caught the medication error, I felt validated that my time at the hospital as an overseer, coordinator, and guardian was paying off—and extremely important for me to continue doing. There would not be many moments when I felt a sense of personal power and value, but this was one time when I did. I felt as if this was a small victory in my battle against cancer, my battle against Ivan's multiple illnesses.

Catching the potentially fatal outcome if Ivan had been given the medication was a big moment for me, and it vindicated my efforts to be in his room every day, especially during nursing shift changes. It vindicated my presence and redeemed me for my prior deplorable actions—or so I tried to convince myself.

After twenty-one days of being in the hospital, Ivan's weight loss impacted his jaw. He was unable to wear his dentures any longer, and this greatly affected his physical appearance and added to feelings of despair for both of us. It felt like our fingers were sliding, losing their grip on a rope line as we looked down into an abyss. He seemed to be sliding backward, and we both were trying to hold on to any rope we could that would lift us out of this nightmare.

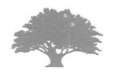

Chapter 17

Going Home

10/21/2003   11:17 p.m.
To: Health Watch Group   (46 people in group)
Subject: Ivan—Update
From: Alison

Hello,

It's Alison again. This is a hard email to write and all of us [mom, Sara and I] have mixed emotions about the latest situation. Today was a tough day. We waited until 4:00 p.m. to speak with the doctor… about his prognosis etc.

Dad made the decision today that he was coming home. This is against what the doctor recommends. The doctor does not think he will survive at home… The main reason is because dad is still not able to process the amount of food needed to fight the cancer. He is still at 50% and needed to be at 100% before leaving the hospital. Therefore, we don't know what the next few days will bring…but dad explained to mom that this is what he wants. He is aware of this and he wants to be home and for us to respect that.

So we are doing everything we can to make home comfortable for him...

We will keep you posted on any news/changes. Please pray for dad for him to be able to process his food and put meat on his bones to fight the cancer... for peace and for the pain to stop. We love all of you and will be in touch soon.

Ivan's strong desire to return home became a new twist in this journey. He was restless and fearful and did not want to fight this fight in the hospital. He had summoned me to sit beside his hospital bed as he told me what he wanted. He believed I could help him more at home than I could at the hospital. He felt my home care would change his health situation and that, with my help, he had a better chance of survival there.

This was extremely scary to me because I felt as if I had the weight of his life in my hands—and *only* my hands. No one lived nearby who could help. Having Ivan at home meant I would be on call 24/7. While Ivan was in the hospital, I was able to take a break from his illness. Having him home meant no breaks from the intensity

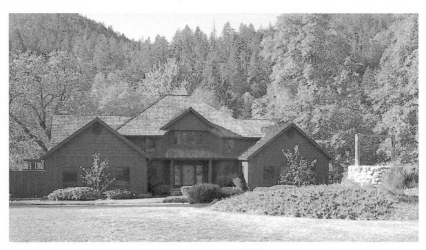

Our home in 2002

of his health issues. I wouldn't be able to get away from the cancer. If something went wrong, it would be my fault—not the hospital's.

We met with his oncologist about his decision to go home, and she did not agree. She felt his condition remained too fragile for me to provide the proper care from home, but she finally agreed after a brief conversation with Ivan. She set up a home health nurse who would visit Ivan at home once a week. The nurse would check Ivan's progress each week, as well as provide a hotline for me, should I have any concerns or problems.

There was so much that needed to be done before he came home. As I thought about the care at home, I thought of his feeding tube, his medicine, his toes, his bedsores, his baths, his mouth sores, his oxygen, and his basic bodily functions. I would need to do it all. My heart raced with those thoughts. I wanted to tell him no and deny his request. The fact that his physician was worried about his care was even more frightening to me, but I decided to honor his request and did not tell him how afraid I was about being placed in this role. I held my reservations inside and started the process of preparing the house.

I found a medical supply place that allowed people to check out medical supplies, and I obtained a bedpan, oxygen cart, wheelchair, walker, and other items the nurses had recommended we have on hand. At the store, I purchased mouth swabs, wound-care supplies, and sheepskin padding for the bed (to help his bedsores).

There were numerous other sundries I needed to buy before he came home that would be needed to treat the various conditions and properly care for him. Ivan felt I could help save him, not the nurses, and I began to believe this too. After all, I had come to fear some of the hospital protocols that I believed put Ivan's life at further risk, and this change meant I could control his care myself. I would become the nursing staff of one—a role that would make me feel empowered and strong.

I was a great organizer, and this was my moment to put those skills to use. Ivan had as many as ten different medications that had to be administered at different times of day. Then there were the tube feedings every three hours and measuring for residual (as the nurses had instructed me) before I dispensed the liquid. If I administered the liquid too quickly or incorrectly, Ivan would throw up, and the process would be unsuccessful. Then I would have to wait another three hours before I could try again. I knew from experience that if I administered the liquid too slowly, Ivan would become irritated and uncomfortable with the position he needed to maintain. I knew this would be a delicate balancing act.

Ivan's toes and feet needed to be massaged daily to prevent the spread of the gangrene. His bedsores needed to be dressed and the healing ointment applied three times a day. The oxygen tubes needed to be checked and the tank monitored twice a day. The sores in his mouth needed constant lubrication with mouth swabs, and he would need to be driven back and forth to the hospital's cancer center each day for his radiation treatment.

The right side of Ivan's face gave the appearance of being pulled down, and the doctors informed me that they believed he'd had a stroke at some point. This meant I needed to watch him closely, to be sure I immediately called 911 should he experience another stroke while under my home care. This also meant that I needed to take his blood pressure twice a day.

When I arrived home and wheeled Ivan into the house, we were greeted by Alison, Kye, and my mom. They had decided to drive up from California to help Ivan and me. Our homecoming was awkward because Ivan was terribly weak and did not feel like greeting people. I didn't look or feel in the least bit strong. I was scared—scared about the new regimen I needed to follow, scared about having my family witness everything I did, and scared that I might make a mistake.

Yet, here were three welcoming people at the back door, watching us as I wheeled Ivan into the house. They greeted us with smiles rather than words and looked at us with sad eyes. As we entered the house, Ditto immediately reacted to Ivan. She jumped back from the wheelchair and cowered into the next room. She cautiously observed Ivan and me from around the corner but made no attempt to get closer and sniff the chair or the man she had once considered her master. She was clearly scared too.

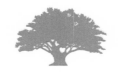

Chapter 18

Family

10/23/2003   9:51 a.m.
To: Health Watch Group   (47 people in group)
Subject: Ivan—Update
From: Alison

Hello everyone,

As you know, Tuesday night was our first night with dad home. Mom was a little apprehensive, but did a GREAT job. We organized all of his meds, feeding schedule, etc. He is very happy to be home in his bed and he can see the river from his room. After talking with dad, we realize this is the best place for him.

Wednesday morning was good for dad too. Jim came to visit dad for a few hours and dad was really happy about that. He can talk—but it's a whisper. This is from the tumor in the throat and he has a strong grip…which is good. And of course he is still making jokes…

He is still going to radiation treatments every day at 11:00 a.m. Once you start they don't recommend you stop. This is week 2 and he will have 6 more *weeks of treatments. After radiation on Wednesday, he was tired and got sick when he returned home. He sleeps most of the time. Even when mom feeds him, he doesn't wake up. He was really nauseated yesterday, so mom was not able to get all of the food in him...*

Wednesday afternoon a Home Health Care nurse came to the house and assessed the house and dad. She checked his vitals etc. and assigned dad a nurse that will come to the house once a week to check dad. This morning, his nurse came to see him and explained to mom that there are several issues to conquer, but she will worry about that and for mom to focus on one at a time. She is available 24 hours a day, which mom is happy about. So today mom is focusing on getting 4 cans of Ensure® in dad. This is the minimum amount and the nurse wants him to try to digest that.

A few of you have asked for dad's prognosis. The doctor said on Wednesday that it's precarious and that she thought he would be back in the hospital in a few days (because of his feeding issue). She explained that he has many issues but that he is a fighter. So you never know. Reality is that he is still fighting strong! We are still struggling with the feedings but working with him on that.

10/26/2003   7:21 p.m.
To: Health Watch Group   (48 people in group)
Subject: Ivan—Update
From: Alison

Hello everyone,

It's Alison again. Sorry we have taken a few days to write. First, thank you so much for the prayers.

They are working and we are pleased and thankful for the amazing family and friends we have!

A few issues developed that we were dealing with—processing food, thrush (in his mouth) and a urinary tract infection. He is still having a hard time processing his food, but we have had nurses here every day working with us to find the right combination and it's definitely improving.

He went to the doctor on Friday and she explained that dad has to maintain his weight. Mom's goal is to feed him 9 cans a day, as many of you now she has a tough time getting 4 cans in him, because he gets really full. The doctor explained to dad that he needs to work hard at trying to let food in his feeding tube. If he does not digest 9 cans a day he will lose 5 lbs. a week. The risk of losing more weight is he will put his other organs into stress mode and overdrive. We don't want this.

Since Friday we have seen improvement. Today he has almost completed 6 cans. We are really excited about that!

As far as his spirits they have really improved. Dad's coloring is a lot better and he is able to walk to the bathroom, living room chair, etc. And today is the first time in a few days he is more awake and watching TV...yeah! He still sleeps a lot but has improved since he has been home, so we are really happy and blessed that he is improving.

Grandma went home on Thursday and Shelby, Ivan's sister came into town yesterday. She will be here for a week to help out. If everything goes well tonight I will be heading home tomorrow. Mom isn't crying as much which is good. She can see the

*improvement in dad and that is making all of us
happy. Now we are just working on getting mom
more sleep. Dad gets up a lot at night so that is making her tired.*

Alison's departure to her home was both distressing and a
relief for me. She had arrived on October 18 and stayed for nine
days. I loved having her with me, having someone to talk to. But
I hated the fact that she was living through these ups and downs
right along with us. It was evident from her email that she felt the
"we" in what was happening with Ivan.

I was in so much self-pity as I adjusted to caring for Ivan at
home that I could not see what Alison was going through. I was
focused on myself—and my belief that no one understood what
I was dealing with. Alison did not go to the doctor's office with
us. She did not help administer the Ensure®. She did not sit with
the nurses as they tried to help me find a way to work with Ivan's
system to process the food. This was all on me.

As I later reflected on Alison, I was angry at myself for placing her in that situation. Alison was there every time I needed
someone to talk to. She was there as a great listener, and she was
a front seat passenger in this ride. I can only imagine how she felt
during those days: watching Ivan struggle and in pain, watching
her mother cry and focus on home care responsibilities. And yet,
in the midst of my day-to-day duties, there was no time for me to
think about her and her pain. I could not be a good wife, a good
nurse, *and* a good mother.

I realize I neglected her during this time, and I've often reflected
on how I could have made her time at the house better and less
painful. I could have talked to her about her own feelings, her
despair, and her fears. I could have wrapped my arms around her
and told her how much I loved her and cherished our moments
together. I could have shared with her what a wonderful young

lady I thought she was and how special she was to me. I could have tried to hug her, the way she was able to hug me, and melt away her shield of strength. Yet, at the time, I could not do any of these things.

Then there was our other daughter, Sara. She had married only two months earlier, moved to San Diego with her new husband, started a job, and enrolled in San Marcus College to finish her final year of college. Her ability to travel to Oregon as frequently as Alison was made difficult because of distance, finances, and her schedule. I can only imagine what emotions Sara must have been feeling, knowing that her sister was with us and she was not, hearing about her father's many health tribulations and being unable to help. The two girls talked daily about what was happening so she could stay involved, even from a distance.

But I did not reach out to Sara to help her deal with her father's failing health either. I left that role to Alison. Looking back, I cannot help but think, *poor Sara*, as much as, *poor Alison*. Sara was left to fend for herself, living in a new area with a new husband, working at a new job, and attending a new school—all the emotional adjustments she was dealing with in addition to her fears and worries about her father's condition.

Unfortunately, as I focused on Ivan's care, I had no capacity to be there for either daughter. I was too consumed by my own emotions and responsibilities to look up and see what my daughters were feeling.

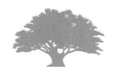

Chapter 19

Process

10/30/2003   2:56 p.m.
To: Health Watch Group   (50 people in group)
Subject: Iva—Update
From: Suzanne

Tomorrow Ivan is scheduled to start the final weeks of radiation—which means he will now have radiation treatments twice a day [10:00 and 4:00]. Since we live far from the center, the group has arranged for us to stay at the Cheney House [a home for families of ill patients at the hospital]. We will stay at the house during the day so Ivan can sleep and I can feed him and tend to his needs. This will be so much easier on him than the drive back and forth.

When Ivan first came home, I was feeding him 2 oz portions every hour on the hour, except between midnight and 5:00. Now I try to feed him every two hours around the clock and his body is accepting up to 8 oz at a time. Although this is a great improvement, he is still only able to process 6 cans a day. We are not giving up though and expect to find more ways to make the feedings work—no matter what time of day. [He has lost another 2 lbs.

The good news is most of the issues he had from his hospital stay have all gone. I am focusing on one or two items in addition to the feedings, which obviously is the critical focus.

I will write again, as time permits, but since most of the day will be spent in town, it will be a little hectic when I get home [caring for the animals, home and setting Ivan up for the night]. I am excited though when I think about the concept that the treatments are almost over and it won't be long before we know if the cancer has been eliminated. Exhausted or not—it's worth the fight and I am in awe over the determination of my husband. I know you would be too if you saw him and saw the fight in his eyes. It's hard to be scared if I focus on "the process" of caring for him and working together to get him well. When I stop to relax or think about the way things are—I cry, but fortunately there isn't a lot of time for this silliness, right?

I wish now I had kept a journal or copied each and every email I received, because it is the small statements and messages from all of you that makes such a difference in my attitude. Thanks.

After being home for about ten days, the second part of the radiation treatment needed to begin. Ivan did not want to stay at the Cheney House (which was a home for families of loved ones who were being treated at the hospital for serious conditions). He preferred to go home in between treatments, so of course, this is what I agreed to do. It was forty-five minutes each way, but this allowed him to rest at home in his own bed.

Everyone had gone home, and I was alone to care for Ivan, the house, and the animals. I had to buy groceries while he was in radiation, clean bathrooms while he slept, and find different ways to take care of other household needs as best I could. I was managing though. The problem was that he seemed to be regressing again.

Ivan complained that he was not feeling well, so the radiologist decided to postpone the double radiation treatment schedule. As a couple of days passed, his breathing seemed labored, and his temperature was beginning to spike. I sensed something was not right again. Ivan would become angry with me if I did not get the pain medicine to him quickly enough, and if I said anything that irritated him, he would scold me and tell me how inadequate I was. These words cut like a knife, and I would often retreat to the back bedroom closet again.

The walk-in closet off the master bedroom became a haven, far from where Ivan was sitting in the living room. As I stood in the dark, holding my face in my hands, I sobbed quietly so he couldn't hear me. I told myself that it was the cancer talking, not Ivan, but this didn't stop me from feeling inadequate and taking in his words that hurt deeply.

I was his savior—the person who was supposed to fix this. If he felt I was not adequate, then what was I? Unfortunately, this was a theme I continued to struggle with. I vowed that I would try harder, do things better, handle my caregiver role more seriously, and be stronger. I would show him and myself that I could succeed in this role.

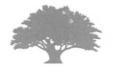

Chapter 20

Food

During the time when Ivan was at home, I focused on what I could do to improve his health. His body's processing of food had consumed my thinking for several weeks. As I strove to increase his body's consumption of the liquid, I did not realize the fluid had begun to create other issues in his system. As other health issues developed, both the oncologist and I finally realized what was happening. The excess was not being processed properly, so this created fluid in his lungs and a blockage in his intestine. I was winning the battle of weight gain and losing the war.

Ivan began to hallucinate, which led the doctors to believe the cancer might have spread to his brain. I refused to share this suspicion with anyone; I just couldn't. Telling anyone this latest information would mean Ivan's fate was doomed; I would be acknowledging the evil illness that had attacked us, and I would be letting it win.

His tests also indicated that there were problems with his gallbladder and liver, which again resulted in the doctor's belief that the cancer was spreading. They had been concerned that the cancer had been stimulated because of the two-week break in treatment while he was in ICU, and it seemed as if they were looking for it in every corner of his body. He had an oncologist, radiologist, nephrologist, phlebologist, pulmonologist, and cardiologist. In other words, they were cancer, radiation, kidney, veins, lung, and heart specialists, to name a few, and they were all looking for signs that the cancer had spread.

I kept thinking of how negative they were being about any change in any little vital sign. I didn't believe they knew if it was the cancer, and yet, they always pointed to the disease as the culprit. I thought they were not trying hard enough to find the real reasons and that they were simply taking the easy way out.

When Ivan became ill and his temperature reached 103, I called the doctor. She told me to bring Ivan into the hospital immediately. This meant that I had to get Ivan from the bedroom into the car by going through the house, across the wooden deck, and into the SUV, which was about fifty yards away. I didn't call 911 because Ivan was adamant that he did not want them to take him.

Although Ivan weighed less than 150 pounds, I could not lift or carry him. I frantically called my neighbor next door, whom I had only briefly met, and she raced over to help me. We slid Ivan onto a desk chair with wheels and rolled him carefully across the various surfaces. It was extremely difficult to roll him and the chair over the rug, across door thresholds, and over uneven ground. He was weak, throwing up blood into a handheld bowl, and visibly in excruciating pain. Somehow, my neighbor and I managed to push and pull him up and into the front passenger seat of the tall SUV. This turned out to be one of the longest drives Ivan and I took to the hospital.

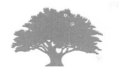

Chapter 21

Readmission

11/04/2003   9:47 a.m.
To: Health Watch Group   (50 people in group)
Subject: Ivan—Update
From: Alison

Hello everyone,

Well, there has been another twist…dad has been readmitted to the hospital.

He was admitted yesterday morning due to severe pain in his right side accompanied by a fever and throwing up. After running a bunch of tests they explained to mom that dad has pneumonia and a severely impacted small intestine. The small intestine is at a stage 8 (at stage 12 it could burst). The doctor explained to mom that they will not release him until this gets cleared up and explained to dad that it might be a couple of days to resolve the issues. On a funny note, mom said when the doctor left the room, dad looked at her and explained that he does not want to be released from the hospital until he is better…and they both laughed.

As you know, dad was supposed to start the double treatments yesterday, but that was postponed because he was not feeling well! However, they will resume the double treatments today. The radiation doctor explained that you cannot pause radiation treatment once you start because it might cause the cancer to spread fast. Therefore, dad must go on with the treatments as planned or he will not be able to start up again.

Mom wanted me to explain that the week ahead looks tough but we will keep you updated with new information as soon as we know anything.

During this hospital stay, I accompanied the transport orderly into the elevator and through several areas to get to the radiation room for Ivan's treatments. Once we returned to his room, I managed any bodily elimination that occurred while Ivan was en route back and forth. I could have waited for a nurse to assist, but they were usually too busy to stop what they were doing to come and assist. Since this was not the job of the transport orderly or the radiation technician, I took care of it each time so that Ivan didn't have to lay in his feces. He was on strong medications, ten in all, and some of these made him sleep through most of the trips to the Radiation Department.

Ivan's mood was changing, as he appeared to accept the fact that he needed help from the medical staff to get well. During his prior hospital stay, he'd shown frustration when the doctor tried to talk to him about being in the hospital, but with this latest admission, he began to let go of trying to control that and allowed others to help him. This was a huge relief to me because I didn't need to fight him about the need to stay in the hospital. I'm not sure if he realized the multitude of processes I had been trying to manage at home or if he accepted that the complexity of his condition required a knowledgeable medical staff, but either way, I was grateful for his change in attitude.

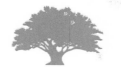

Chapter 22

Roller Coaster Ride

Once again, the roller coaster of health issues ensued. It was déjà vu all over again—the return of issues with Ivan's intestinal tract, his kidneys, his lungs, his blood pressure, and his temperature. It was all happening again, and I felt defeated. The progress we had made at home had been wiped out, erased. As we attempted to plug one hole in the boat, another developed, giving me little time to relax.

As I wrote to friends or informed family, they openly expressed their sadness and worry about the ongoing decline. Ivan became quieter too. Clearly, he realized the magnitude of each issue as it arose, and he stated his disappointment with the backward sliding of his health. When he expressed his own deflated feeling, I felt immensely sad. His strength had helped me stay strong, so without it, I felt disheartened.

> *11/05/2003*　　　　　　　*6:41 p.m.*
> *To: Health Watch Group　(50 people in group)*
> *Subject: Ivan—Update*
> *From: Suzanne*
>
> *Just a quick note to let you know Ivan is doing REALLY well. His lungs are clearing, the intestine*

is improving and they have switched to a different type of Ensure® to help in his processing. The doctor thinks he will be able to go home in a couple of days!

The new days back in the hospital meant a return to the former routine with Ditto, my early morning and late-night schedule, and my oversight of the medical and nursing staff to ensure the right medicines were administered or the proper treatment occurred. I felt more defeated this time as I went through each of these motions. Thoughts of losing Ivan and being alone occurred frequently, and it seemed these fears were consuming me more and more. I tried to suppress these concerns and feelings, but it was becoming more difficult to stuff them down.

11/07/2003   10:46 p.m.
To: Health Watch Group   (50 people in group)
Subject: Ivan—Update
From: Alison

Hello everyone,

We wanted to give you another update, but we're waiting to hear from the doctors today. Dad took a different turn yesterday. He started to really hallucinate and was having conversations that were concerning to mom. The nurses and doctors made a note in dad's file and they are watching him. He also was unable to keep food down yesterday, he was throwing up and it was hard for him to breathe. They increased his oxygen and lowered the amount of food to try and keep some nutrition in his body. He did not want mom to leave his side so she got home late last night and did not sleep well.

That was yesterday's events…today she got to the hospital at 6:00 a.m. She just met with the doctors.

He still has pneumonia and is having dreams but not like yesterday (mom said today he is more alert). His small intestine is still impacted but not as bad as Monday. The pain is less for dad which is a good sign. His blood tests show that his gallbladder and liver numbers have dropped. Therefore, today they are doing an ultra sound to check those organs out. We should know the status later this afternoon. They are continuing to monitor his lungs—he is at a level 3 oxygen. They will be doing an x-ray of his lungs on Sunday. They are also trying to increase his food today to see if he can handle more CCs. Yesterday, he was getting 25 CCs per hour and today they are trying to up it to 50 CCs per hour. To give you an idea there are 30 CCs in one ounce.

Needless to say, every day is a new day. His situation is continuing to be under watch. Now we really understand what the doctor meant when she said his situation was precarious. So on that note...we are not sure when dad will be released from the hospital. As many of you are experiencing with us it changes every day. Just know that we really appreciate all of your thoughts and prayers. We will let you know more as soon as we find out.

The realization that Ivan's health was precarious was more disheartening to me than we stated. When he consumed more Ensure®, his intestines and lungs filled up, but when we backed off the Ensure® and his lungs and intestines improved, he lost the precious weight he needed to fight the cancer. Friends and family must have seen this dilemma. I felt our efforts were futile, and more than ever, an overwhelming sadness was hard to shake off. It had been seven weeks since Ivan entered the hospital the first time, and since that time, our days had been filled with the ups and downs of his failing health.

> *11/10/2003*   *10:38 a.m.*
> *To: Health Watch Group* *(50 people in group)*
> *Subject: Ivan—Update*
> *From: Alison*
>
> *Good morning everyone,*
> *Everything is looking really good! YEAH! Dad is a little tired today but doing a lot better. His lungs are sounding better every day and he is processing his food well. Here is some great news—Dad has gained weight! He weighs 123   The doctor is really pleased with his results.*
> *Dad was given the option today of being able to go home from the hospital. However, he is talking with mom about that. He will continue to have 2 radiation treatments a day which will drain him. So he is thinking he might stay in the hospital a few more days to help increase his strength. We will let you know any changes, but for now things are looking great and he could be home in a few days.*

Alison continued to keep friends and family abreast of Ivan's progress. During my breaks with Ditto, I called Alison and gave her updates. It felt great to talk to her and to be able to share my worries. I hated to return to Ivan's hospital room because the atmosphere was so stressful and sad. I preferred to stay outside with Ditto and walk the perimeter of the hospital grounds.

I had brought a picture of Ivan and me and placed it on the bedside table near his bed to help the cold, sterile room feel homier for him. Often the nurses commented on the happy, healthy picture of us and how it was motivating to them to return Ivan to the man in the picture. But I didn't feel motivated. The picture was a sad reminder of the days gone by and the dreams that retirement were intended to provide. I began to lose faith that we'd ever get back to those dreams.

11/17/2003   *7:07 a.m.*
To: Health Watch Group   *(51 people in group)*
Subject: Ivan —Update
From: Suzanne

I am so sorry I haven't written for a while. The news became so difficult to hear let alone write; I crawled into my usual shell and stayed there. But I'm better now and will try to update all of you who have been eager to hear the update.

1. *Alison had written that Ivan had gained weight— as the nurses had told us, but this was incorrect. The nurse who took the weight did not calibrate the bed correctly. He actually had lost weight [as of Friday he weighed 117]. But I believe WE ALL needed to hear some good news that day—so we heard what we needed to keep going.*

2. *Ivan's pneumonia became even worse than before on last Thursday. The doctor believes that since his tongue can't swallow or perform the regular functions, his stomach liquid is traveling into his lungs when he sleeps thus creating pneumonia. They have stopped the stomach feeds and put him on TPN [a nutritional substance that is put into his blood instead]. The positive is his body LOVES this stuff and is responding really well.*

3. *His circulation in his legs is greatly reduced and he's been breaking down cholesterol deposits into the lower leg and feet. This has been painful as they travel to smaller veins and get stuck. They have also created blood clots in some of the toes which have now turned into gangrene. This news was particularly disheartening for Ivan [and therefore me] to hear. They want him sitting up and walking as much as he can take and you need to know THAT IS JUST WHAT HE IS DOING. He's amazing. They hope that the body handles the toe condition on its own or they will have to remove the affected toes.*

All in all, we have been sad, as I said—but last night when I left the hospital, Ivan and I talked about this coming week and the focus on the finish line. Wednesday should be our last double-treatment day [possibly Thursday if they think his system can stand an extra dose]. The doctor said he may be able to go home to complete his recovery from all that he has going on.

I need to go now—running late this morning and I want to be there for the doctor visit you know.

The radiation treatment consisted of two parts: the first part was one weekly dosage and the second part entailed two doses a day for several weeks. Although we were focused on completing the radiation regimen, our true worry was whether or not the treatment had been successful. We would not learn the results until several weeks after the treatment was finished, when they would run another CT scan of the area, so I was anxious about the results of our efforts. The sad eyes of the radiologist were imprinted in my mind. He constantly expressed his concern over

Ivan's health issues and tried to increase the dose as much as possible. Seeing the physician's concern caused me to wonder if he knew that the treatment was in vain but he didn't want to tell us. I interpreted dark shadows in every corner, and even the slightest comment from a nurse or physician made me wonder if they were keeping something from us. I worried that they knew Ivan would not survive, and this added to my stress.

11/21/2003   *10:43 a.m.*
To: Health Watch Group   *(51 people in group)*
Subject: Ivan—Update
From: Alison

Good morning,

Mom asked me to send the latest update because she really wants everyone to pray with us...As you all know dad has difficulty swallowing and is unable to have Ensure® anymore. They moved him to TPN which is food through an IV.

Here is the deal. Dad was supposed to be released today but this will NOT happen because the TPN IV was not approved through Medicare. This means that it would cost $550 per day if he came home with TPN. As you all know dad is very intelligent and explained to the doctor that Medicare will be losing money with him in the hospital than at home and that this should be approved.

They are going to be performing a test today that takes 6 hours to see if he can qualify for it to be covered by Medicare. It's a barium test. They will put barium in his feeding tube and if he is able to process it before 6 hours he will not qualify and will not be released. However, if it takes his body longer than 6 hours he will qualify and be released from the hospital with the TPN on Monday or Tuesday morning.

This is what both mom and dad really want. Yes, he does have pneumonia and other things wrong but he really wants to be home for Thanksgiving. Monday will be 3 weeks that he has been back in the hospital and he does not want to stay there anymore. So we are asking that all of you pray with us for this test to work!

Now...

If his body does process the barium before 6 hours this means they will have to put another tube in dad that will go directly to his small intestine. If this needs to be done the procedure would happen next week. After this procedure he would have to stay in the hospital for one week to make sure his body accepts the new tube. The doctor explained if the tube is rejected they will remove it and come up with another alternative. However, if his body accepts it they will release him the week after Thanksgiving.

A lot of 'Ifs' so that is why we really want to have everyone praying that this first procedure works. Dad and mom are both depressed/saddened by the news today! and so are Sara and myself...Dad really wants to go home and the doctor's informed mom and dad today that he has the same chance of recovery at home because he will be sent home with antibiotics, hospital bed, etc. Therefore, all of your prayers and support is greatly appreciated.

The hospital regimen took its toll on Ivan too. The radiation treatments had been completed, but the battle with his lungs, heart, and new bedsores were exhausting to both of us. He spoke very little, due to the painfulness of his throat, but when he talked, he talked about being at home. That's why the new test to check his bodily function was frustrating and sad. We found ourselves hoping he had issues with his functions so he could be released. This was a catch-22 for us. How crazy it seemed that we were praying for yet another issue that we would have to manage. But Ivan seemed to find strength with the thought of getting home, and I needed his strength more than ever before. I was reaching new lows emotionally and finding it difficult to keep any positive thoughts going.

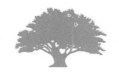

Chapter 23

Home Again

11/24/2003   *12:16 p.m.*
To: Health Watch Group *(51 people in group)*
Subject: Ivan—Update
From: Alison

Hello everyone,
    Just wanted to let you know that I got a call from mom; dad will be coming home this afternoon! Thank you for all of your thoughts and prayers.

Alison and Kye drove from Sacramento the day before Thanksgiving, bringing with them a full dinner from Safeway. We did our best to set the table in a festive fashion, and with a fire in the fireplace, we made the house as warm and welcoming as possible. We had a lot to be grateful for! This was our first Thanksgiving in our new home since retiring, and it truly was special. Ivan was home, he was safe, we were with one of our daughters, and life was getting better. I felt relieved, relaxed, and loved.

After the many days of heartbreak and heartache, this day felt like a wonderful reprieve. We were able to convince ourselves that life was good again, and the charade seemed to work. Cancer was not in the room with us. Ivan was not the sick man he had been just days before in the hospital bed. He dressed in nice slacks and a sweater, and he wore a smile. He sat in his chair while we ate at the table because he could not swallow or eat regular food. But it did not matter. He was with us.

I was grateful and relieved that Alison and Kye were with Ivan and me too. They were our companions, and having them with us helped us to feel safe. I had support. I relaxed with their presence because they had bought happiness at the store and placed it on our table of pain and melancholy. The Thanksgiving dinner was a symbolic moment of our pretense about cancer. It was proof that it had not divided our love; it had not stripped our family of our foundation; it was not winning.

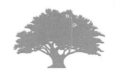

Chapter 24

More than Cancer

The term "holidays" typically conjures up a feeling of fun, happy moments with friends and family for me. That was anything but what I felt during these days. Ivan's mood swings, from tearful exchanges to declarations of his strong determination to beat this illness, were exhausting. I walked on eggshells, not sure what to expect from him, yet wanting to support whatever he was feeling.

> *12/03/2003   11:43 a.m.*
> *To: Health Watch Group   (51 people in group)*
> *Subject: Ivan—Update*
> *From: Suzanne*
>
> *Hi,*
>
> *First, I apologize for not updating you all sooner. The schedule isn't bad now that we're at home, it just seems like I never make the time needed to work at the computer.*
>
> *Ivan has continued to improve—note: his oxygen was taken off Monday! His lungs are great and the doctor is really pleased with his progress. Yeah for him!*

Most of his other issues are continuing to improve, with the exception of the toes and the kidneys. We are scheduled to see a surgeon for the toes and the kidney doctor about the embolic clots in the next two weeks. To help you get an idea of "what's next" here is the timing:

1. *Meet with the doctor about possible removal of toes [in 2 weeks]*

2. *Meet with kidney doctor about possible effects on kidney as result of embolic deposits that are releasing in the blood [in 2 weeks]*

3. *Meet with doctor about possible need [or not] for insert of new tube into small intestine [in 1 week]*

4. *Meet with Radiation doctor to run last tests to see if they got all of the cancer [in 5 weeks]*

5. *Meet with Throat surgeon if surgery is next [if they did not get it all]. [in 6 weeks]*

Between now and Christmas we will be meeting with the various doctors I mentioned; and taking one day at a time. As you know, he has a long way to go—but he looks great right now!

We feel blessed to be home, to have survived the various ordeals at the hospital and we fell blessed for the friends and family in our lives. Ivan has been very melancholy about this aspect—but that's to be expected. The doctor told him to cry when he felt like it and get angry when he felt like it too. That it is all part of the healing process for serious illnesses, so he's been doing good on this aspect too...

Hope I've answered some of your questions about his health right now. And, thank you all so much for your prayers. What a powerful group of people we know. It is our one comment EVERY DAY.

The more time that passed and Ivan's illness progressed, the more we needed the services of a speech therapist. His throat had become strained from the radiation, and he, therefore, needed assistance to learn to speak and enunciate clearly. The therapist came to the house once a week and worked with Ivan for about an hour each time. Listening from another room was heart-wrenching for me, as I heard Ivan try to repeat the words directed by the therapist. He was barely able to repeat them clearly in the beginning, but after weeks of practice, his speech began to improve.

12/10/2003   *8:50 p.m.*
To: Health Watch Group (51 people in group)
Subject: Ivan—Update
From: Suzanne

Still good news comin'...I thought I would state that right away, since I understand some of you cautiously open my emails   and for a while, you had good reason.

Ivan has returned the wheel chair and he is walking a lot now, very stable. He uses the walker for 'insurance' but his skinny legs are getting stronger.

The pneumonia is gone! Yeah baby. And our list of issues is down to a small handful.

He weighs 113.4 lbs.   but he looks great.

I've nicknamed him "The Pink Panther" [cartoon] since he has such skinny arms—skinny legs - skinny butt—and he is feisty...which makes him laugh [so please don't think ill of me for teasing him].

The speech therapist said Ivan is progressing amazingly well and he believes he will be able to eat and drink again soon. "soon" means months—not weeks—but that's great news because it means we will forgo the surgery to have a tube inserted in his small intestine....[yeahhhhhhhhhh....and the crowd goes wild]

Next Tuesday we see the surgeon about possible removal of his toes and on that same day we see the kidney doctor about the status of possible clotting in his kidneys. We are putting our energy into that day begin a great day. No bad news; Just opportunities.

Well, as you probably can tell, I'm a little silly tonight. Good news and lack of sleep will do it every time. But I won't APOLOGIZE...shocker...haha

Oh—best news of this email: We are going to be grandparents in August! Sara and Kevin are expecting! Ivan cried when Sara called. He was truly overcome with emotion...as we should be.

That's it for now. Thanks, as always, for being there for us!

At that point, I felt anxious and disheartened. I tried to manage each health condition, but I believed it was only a matter of time before another string of bad news was announced. I didn't trust the possibility that we were climbing out of the horrific hole of sadness. While the days were filled with managing appointments and Ivan's bodily needs, these activities allowed me to maintain a good front and veil my emotional apprehensions.

The care for Ivan had not become lighter, even if some of his conditions were improving. I struggled to envision better days for us in the future, and the announcement of Sara's pregnancy made me worry about whether or not Ivan would be around to see the birth of our first grandchild. This concern was what I believed he felt, too, when he broke down and cried, but neither one of us said anything aloud. My hope was beginning to dissipate, but I did not share this with others.

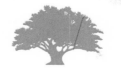

Chapter 25

Brother Buzz

My brother Frank is my eldest brother and has always been protective and caring. He was there for me when I was going through a divorce; he was there for me when I was involved in family litigation; he was there for me each time I went through painful moments; and after Ivan became ill, he wanted to be there for me again. I called him "Brother Buzz" after a children's TV character from our childhood.

Frank was a golfing buddy of Ivan's, and the two men played pool whenever he and his wife, Kathy, came over for dinner. We had lived twenty minutes away from each other in Fremont, California, where Frank and I had grown up. Ivan and Frank teased each other constantly, in a fun-loving way, and you could see the close bond they shared when you watched them interact.

It had been five months since Ivan was first diagnosed with cancer, back in July, and two months since he'd been hospitalized in critical condition in October. Frank was very concerned about Ivan's health, but he was a high school teacher and a swim coach raising a family of his own in the Bay Area. As much as he longed to drive up to Oregon and spend time with us, his work, family, and the illness of our stepfather kept him from being able to do so.

The six-month period from June to November had been horrible for him. Cancer had played a major role in his life once more. Although it had been almost thirty years since cancer destroyed the life of our father back in 1974, it had taken the life of a close friend the previous August and struck again shortly after by ending the life of our stepfather in September. It seemed to be trying once more to destroy someone he loved by attacking his sister's husband—his friend.

He was distraught about all the news he heard from Alison and felt compelled to drive up with Kathy from Northern California and spend a week of their vacation with us. Frank worked around the property, nonstop. His nervous energy helped to repair sprinklers, replace worn-out lights, mow lawns, trim bushes, and rake leaves. The six-and-a-half-acre property was daunting, but he never complained.

Kathy cooked and prepared our meals, picked up around the house, and took care of many of the inside chores. This allowed me to be with Ivan and take care of his health needs. They were a godsend, and I loved having them near me.

The week passed quickly, and when the time came for them to leave, I was devastated. I enjoyed their company, but most of all, I wanted their companionship. The house had felt full with them there. The sounds of the mower outside, the pots and pans in the kitchen, as well as the voices and busy activities, made the house come alive. I cringed at the thought of being alone again.

As we walked to their car and said goodbye, I held back the tears that were trying to burst forth. I did not want them to feel bad that they could not stay longer; I wanted them to feel happy that they had contributed to our household needs and supported me. I was so proud to have such a loving brother and sister-in-law. We hugged for several minutes, and before he got into his car, Frank said, "Take care of my good friend Ivan." My heart jumped into my stomach. It felt like he expected me to save Ivan—to do all I could to give him the proper care so he would survive this illness.

I adored my brother. I would do anything for him. But how could I tell him that his simple statement was daunting and gut-wrenching? How could I tell him how scared I was to be left alone to battle an illness that was a relentless adversary?

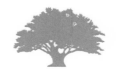

Chapter 26

Mixed Emotions

12/16/2003   *9:28 p.m.*
To: Health Watch Group   *(53 people in group)*
Subject: Ivan—Update
From: Suzanne

The results of the doctor visits are mixed:

1. *Surgeon: He says Ivan has Peripheral Artery disease and he doesn't want to remove the toes that are gangrene because he is concerned that the foot would not heal, due to poor circulation in the leg. He wants to see if there is a blockage in one of the main arteries near the abdomen. If so—he said we will discuss our options later.*

   Monday is an ultra sound to see if they find anything. If they can't see anything with the ultrasound—then they will insert dye and conduct an arteriogram after the holiday. [the arteriogram provides the doctor with a 'map' of the arteries based on a series of x-rays & dye] We won't use the dye as our first option—since the kidneys react negatively to the dye that is used in these procedures.

2. *Renal Doctor: Although the Oncologist expressed concern that the kidney may be affected by the embolic spillage or blockage, the kidney doctor wants to wait and see if they can bring Ivan's blood pressure down through an increase in the medicine. [His pressure has been very high over the past few days]. She also stated that if the pressure continues to increase and nothing else manifests itself as the cause then she will work with the surgeon on injecting the dye in a manner that will also show the arteries to the kidneys.*

I'm sure this must be confusing—since I find it hard to state the facts without a drawn out explanation, so forgive me.

I guess it's fair to say "good news" that the toes will not be removed. I know Ivan is happy about that—regardless of the reason. [He told the doctor that it's his "pivot foot for golf and he doesn't want to affect his swing because he plans on golfing again".]

I think the best comment I can make was told to me by my daughter Alison, and that is that "we can't get upset about the possible blockage because we don't know what options will be available to us in order for this matter to be resolved." So we will continue to keep a positive view!

Take care and we wish you all a wonderful holiday season with your friends and family. Give a hug to yourself...from us!

Christmas—a holiday that is packed with emotions of joy, hope, and peace—was upon us. This one was the opposite of any I had known in my life. Ivan and I were alone. The girls could not drive up from California, and friends and family were busy with their own holiday events and plans. I convinced myself that it would be great to be alone, to be together, but I was wrong. The days leading up to Christmas and the holiday itself were almost unbearable.

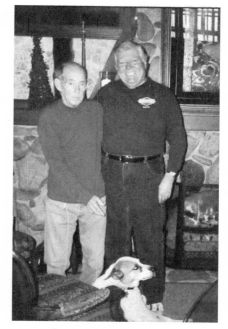

Ivan and his friend Bill

One of Ivan's close personal friends, whom he had known since early childhood, drove up from Southern California to visit Ivan. I helped dress Ivan in clothes that hung loosely on him. While I was dressing him, Ivan stepped over to glance at himself in the mirror. He gasped out loud, and I quickly turned toward him, not sure what had happened. He was motionless, staring in the mirror as tears welled up in his eyes. I had forgotten that Ivan had not used a mirror over these past several months. He did not know how much his physical appearance had changed; he still saw himself in the same way he had looked six months earlier. I rubbed his shoulder and continued to dress him, neither one of us saying anything.

Bill had been worried about his dear friend and wanted to see him and offer assistance and support. But he was devastated when he saw Ivan. Although I had been watching Ivan's physical appearance change gradually, Bill was not prepared for this. He was visibly shaken and struggled to make small talk. He fumbled with words as he asked how Ivan was doing.

I served a meager plate of crackers and cheeses, which were stale, and put a fire in the fireplace to try to create a comfortable setting. We visited for a couple of hours until Ivan informed Bill that he was too tired to stay up any longer. Bill graciously understood and prepared to leave. He asked if he could have a picture taken with Ivan. Ivan agreed. We sat Ditto in front of the two men, but she would not stay, careful not to lean toward Ivan.

As I walked Bill to his car and thanked him for coming, he looked into my eyes and told me, "Take care of my best friend." His voice cracked, and he continued to tell me he did not want to lose Ivan, so he needed me to do everything I could to help him. My heart sank again. How could I tell him how difficult this situation had become and how unbearably heavy his statement made me feel—the pressure to keep my husband alive, to conquer cancer? My heart felt like it was in my throat, and I could not respond, except with an accepting nod. I did not feel anger or resentment toward him for his request. After all, he cared deeply about Ivan and simply wanted him to survive. I was sad, though, because I couldn't help but feel inadequate against this formidable enemy. And I couldn't tell Bill what my real fear was—that I didn't feel I could save Ivan.

On Christmas Day, Ivan was melancholy and asked me to lay next to him in the bed. He had been remembering better times with our kids and the dreams of a joyous retirement. As we held each other, he sobbed and repeatedly told me how sorry he was—for his illness, for his depression at Christmastime, for not buying me a gift, for not planning a more celebratory day, for everything. He could not stop crying, and neither could I.

I was exhausted and drained. Christmas had always been a happy time of planning dinners, organizing gatherings, exchanging gifts, attending parties, and experiencing other special moments that we declared family traditions. I had done none of these things in preparation for this Christmas, so I felt responsible for Ivan's depression.

Each of our twenty-four prior Christmas holidays had been special, and they'd made me feel important. I felt I had been the catalyst for creating incredibly fond memories for our family. This Christmas was hardly that. I felt inadequate as a mother and a wife. I had not sent any gifts to the kids. I had not shopped or made gifts for anyone, not even for Ivan. I was holding Ivan in my arms, crying, and I realized that this would be the only memory I created. I had allowed myself to become a victim of cancer, and I could not shift my mind to stop the self-pity it was creating in me. Admittedly, this was not a proud moment for me, as Ivan cried because of his feelings of guilt. Feeling my own sense of guilt, I continued to cry too.

Wanting to find a way to rectify this situation, I thought of an idea that I felt my kids might like. I had bought a vintage Christmas journal the year before, but I had not used it. I thought it would be wonderful if each of us wrote about our Christmas apart, creating a family memory that would bring us all together in one journal. I thought if Ivan and I were experiencing a lonely, sad holiday, it would be something we could look back on to celebrate the success of overcoming this difficult time. I also thought the girls might be experiencing sadness because we could not be together, and the journal could be a chance to express how they were feeling so they could eventually look back at what they'd written and celebrate overcoming their difficulties too.

I was excited about the idea because it felt like a cure to the melancholy. I believed the gift of expressing our feelings would be more meaningful than any items we might have purchased. Deep down, I thought that this journal would help the girls to understand what Ivan and I were going through—how hard our life had become and how lonely it was without them near us. I also thought using the journal to express my feelings in writing would be easier than trying to share my feelings in person.

I wrote about our loneliness, our embrace on the bed, and our shared tears. I wrote about receiving a large box from my sister, who had sent several small wrapped gifts for Ivan and me to open. I wrote the lyrics of "Have Yourself a Merry Little Christmas," and I ended my journal entry with the hope that next Christmas we would have a new entry from each of us that would reflect how our lives had turned around.

I sent the book to Alison and asked her and Kye to write their own entry and then pass it on to Sara so that she and Kevin could do the same. Ultimately, we would have an annual journal of Christmas memories that would allow us to see where we had been and all that we had to cherish, whether we were together or apart for the holiday.

I thought it was a great idea, but it failed. Alison was so devastated by the entry I had written, she refused to write in the book. My feeble attempt to create incredibly fond memories was dashed. Unintended, I had only given my girls more pain. Afterward, I felt horrible and guilty for not having had more sensitivity to their feelings and emotions. While I was experiencing the cancer that had attached itself to our family, so were my daughters—a fact that I had not considered.

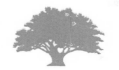

Chapter 27

My Sister

The one bright light in our Christmas holiday came in the form of a large brown box sent by my sister, Lynn. It was full of surprises for Ivan and me that offered a few moments of delight and lightheartedness.

Lynn, who is the second oldest, is a loving, caring, and kind-hearted person. Being four years younger than Lynn, I adored her all through my childhood. From as far back as I could remember, I felt my sister was beautiful, smart, and perfect in my eyes. I believed she could do no wrong, and I looked up to her all through school. She was a straight-A student who had also learned from our mom how to sew and cook, and she was a great cook. When we were growing up, Mom often asked her to help in the kitchen. I, on the other hand, was not like my sister in the kitchen. In fact, my single experience with cooking revealed why my parents relied on my sister when Mom needed help.

I was about nine years old when my mom asked me to cook hotdogs and beans one night for my two brothers. The rest of the family would be out that night. I had always observed my mother cooking for an hour before we were called to the dinner table, so I started both food items with this in mind. After the dutiful hour had passed, I called my brothers to the table and attempted to spoon the beans onto their plates. The beans were so stiff and dense that they could not be scooped without pushing them off the spoon. They formed a hard mound on our plates. The hotdogs were split and swollen beyond recognition. The skin barely held the hotdogs together. My brothers laughed out loud and joked about the disaster I'd created as they left the table without even taking a bite.

When my parents came home, the two of them reenacted the whole story to my mother. They pointed at me as they held their sides, wiped away tears of laughter, and joked about the woeful site on their dinner plates. My mom only stared at me and shook her head. I was heartbroken. Sadly for me, my brothers often retold this story when they wanted to share a good laugh with their friends or other family members. Eventually, I was able to appreciate the humor in it too.

As Lynn and I grew older, we spent time together sporadically. After she moved out to attend college, our lives seemed to travel on somewhat different paths. We each had careers in very different fields, and our marriages and children did overlap. But no matter how time passed, we always managed to reignite our connection when we got together. We would tell stories, joke, and laugh as we reminisced about our childhood.

Unfortunately, after my stepfather was diagnosed with lung cancer, his health seemed to deteriorate quickly, and my mom was not prepared for the care he required. Lynn lived close to Mom and John, so she was able to help with many of the logistics for my mom, including preparing dinner for her and running errands.

Although I knew my mom was probably going through many of the same caregiver issues that I was experiencing, I did not call her and talk to her about it. I left those conversations to my sister and oldest brother. I was spent emotionally and didn't have more to give. I also kept my own nightmare to myself since I knew they had plenty to manage already. After John's diagnosis, my mom had expressed her disappointment for not being able to travel to

Oregon to be with Ivan and me, so I didn't want to say anything that might contribute to feelings of guilt on our behalf.

When my mom told me that hospice was setting up their home so John could be home with her, I realized her time with John was limited. I knew that the presence of hospice meant John had only a few months to live. I'm sure mom knew this, too, but neither one of us spoke about a timeline, nor did we talk about the fear she must have been feeling. Since my sister was there, I told myself that she would be there for our mom. Although I felt guilty for making this choice, I wasn't emotionally or physically capable of doing anything more to support her.

Lynn stayed with Mom during the final hours of John's life, which I later learned were filled with painfully traumatic gestures and movements, as John's body attempted to stop the agonizing suffering. I was spared these vivid, emotional moments; Lynn was not. She endured these sorrowful days alongside my mom, offering her as much support as possible.

As I looked at the large brown box my sister had sent, delivered by UPS just before Christmas, I was in awe of her generosity and love. Not only was Lynn's time consumed with supporting our mom, but she was also a single parent who was managing her own children and household, as well as a job. I marveled at her capacity to do something so thoughtful for the two of us. How she ever had time to send Ivan and me a box full of gifts at Christmas, I'll never know.

And neither Ivan nor I could have conceived of what was hidden inside. When I cut through the box, my chest felt like someone was standing on it. A treasure trove of individually wrapped gifts lay inside. As I opened each present, Ivan and I stared at each other. There were small gifts of winter gloves and scarves, as well as other items selected especially for each one of us. My sister's thoughtfulness was truly overwhelming and, in that moment, I had a deeper understanding of her capacity for love.

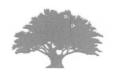

Chapter 28

New Year

1/03/2004   10:30 a.m.
To: Health Watch Group (51 people in group)
Subject: Ivan—Update
From: Suzanne

Happy New Year.

 It has been a long time since I wrote- sorry.

 On Christmas Eve Ivan's blood count fell again, so he had a transfusion of 3 units that took all day. It helped though, and he began to feel better the next day. [He had been ill with fever, etc. and they believe his kidney is not functioning properly right now to produce the substance needed to trigger the production of red blood cells. So, each week, he will now get a shot to help this along.

 We heard back from the last test on the Peripheral Artery Disease—and his right thigh artery is almost completely blocked. The left side moderately blocked. We will address the 'next step' [putting a stint to open the area] after we know what is happening on the cancer.

Although we spent Christmas alone [with each other] the girls came up for the New Years' weekend and that was great. We also have had various friends drive up and visit Ivan since Thanksgiving and that has been good for his spirits. My brother and his wife came up for a week and she cooked while he did chores around the property. Ivan was restless and depressed, but the doctor told him this was normal for the severity of his illness and the holiday season. He is doing better now!

I'll try to outline 'what's next' so you can understand where our prayers are right now:

1/7- Ivan has a CT scan to see if they got all of the cancer. Our doctor visit before Christmas was not very hopeful as the lymph node is still hard and sore but he admitted we had a couple of weeks before the test, so things could improve.

1/8- Doctor apt to learn the results and find out if he will need surgery. If they did not get all of the cancer then the doctor told us he will send Ivan down to UCSF for the surgery, since he is considered 'high risk' with all of the other issues [kidney, heart, pneumonia, loss of weight, etc.] He told us Ivan would have the surgery right away, so we may be in the Bay Area in a week or so. We will learn more once we know the results.

If they got it all, we begin a follow up maintenance program and move on to the next issue to resolve.

Health Issue Triage:

- *Cancer [if surgery is needed]*

- *Artery Disease [procedure to insert stint]*

- *Throat—increase muscle control of throat and*

tongue in order to eat and drink again [this will help return the weight]

- *Neck Surgery—arthritis found to be severe around the top of the spine and hampering the nerve area. Surgery needed to clear this area to avoid future paralysis.*

- *Gangrene Toes—removal remains an option only if the body does not discard the affected area naturally.*

Although the holidays were tough [with daily issues and the emotions evoked at this time of year], we are grateful to be together, fighting this illness and finding new ways to enjoy the beauty in each day.

May you be as blessed with friends and family in your lives as we are!

We will write again once we know the results, I promise.

It was a blessing to have the girls join us for New Years. Kevin, Sara's husband, was unable to take time off from work, but we flew Sara up, and Kye and Alison joined us as well. The girls were happy to spend time with us, and Alison encouraged me to inform others about the status of Ivan's health, but the task seemed daunting. The number of issues Ivan was facing felt overwhelming when I listed them for the email. Managing them one at a time felt easier than seeing them stacked up.

I felt relieved to have the girls close. Ivan slept most of the time, but just having the rest of us sitting around the dinner table, sharing stories and laughing, seemed a welcomed break from the pressure of my caregiver tasks.

1/05/2004   *8:30 a.m.*
To: Alison
Subject: Ivan—Update
From: Suzanne

Hi babe.

    We dropped off Sara at 6:45 and the weather is good so I believe her flights will be easy for her today.

    With her departure, came the realization that we are alone again…you're gone, Frank's gone…and we both felt incredibility sad. Don't cry though cause I know we will see you guys soon. I will stay busy today so as to get through the day and then I'll get to call you to hear your peppy voice and find out how Kye's first day went.

Alison and Kye had experienced a significant amount of change since their marriage in June 2003. They'd moved into their first home in Sacramento, Alison had begun work at a local insurance brokerage firm, and Kye had started a new job in January 2004.

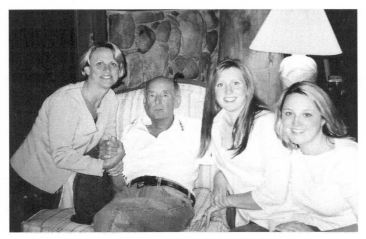

Me, Ivan, Sara and Alison – Fall 2003

They were excited to begin their new life together and build a family. The pressure of performing well on their new jobs, while staying involved with Ivan's and my needs, was a struggle for both. Alison talked about wanting to spend time with me and helping out, but she worried about the impact of taking time off.

Kye was a quiet supporter of Alison's need to be with us. Prior to Ivan's illness, he had enjoyed talking to Ivan about work and life issues, and he'd relied heavily on Ivan's guidance and support. The thought of losing Ivan was difficult for Kye to comprehend, and he seemed to need to keep his distance from us and his emotions guarded.

1/09/2004   *8:47 a.m.*
To: Health Watch Group   *(59 people in group)*
Subject: Ivan—Update
From: Suzanne

The doctor cancelled the appointment since we did not have the test but he later called last night and told us the plan will be:

1. Monday—Ivan will have the MRI

2. Following Monday—we will meet with the throat doctor to discuss results. He said he may also take a biopsy of the tongue area to see if the cancer is gone there.

3. Based on the MRI and biopsy we will discuss our options and possible travel to SF

Although I am disappointed that we have to wait, I believe the time is given so Ivan can continue to get strong and heal more and more...so...we're not sad.

We'll write again after the doctor apt [in two weeks]

Back at home, and on my own, my day consisted of household chores, routine care of the dog and cat, and the constant care of Ivan. I did not cook regular meals for myself. Instead, my meals consisted of quick, microwavable foods, such as pot pies or soups. My physical appearance began to change because of my food choices, and this included an increase in my weight. It especially showed in my stomach, hips, thighs, and arms. Having once sported a slender size four, I could easily slip into a size fourteen.

Although I had always been careful about my attire and how I looked outwardly, this, too, had changed. I constantly felt tired, and my face looked drawn. I no longer bothered with makeup or hair styling. I didn't care how I looked. I didn't have the desire or energy to care. I selected loose, baggy tops and long pants. These helped to hide the figure that had lost its slender shape.

Even though I rarely slept or exercised, my health was other-wise fine, but it honestly didn't matter to me anymore. My focus was on Ivan and keeping his needs met—helping him to get well—it was not on me. This was my role, to care for and support Ivan, and with each passing day, I felt more in control and stronger than ever because I believed I was providing the care Ivan needed. My own needs seemed inconsequential; his needs, and me meeting those needs, were significant and what mattered most to me.

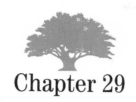

Chapter 29

Shattered

1/13/2004   4:28 p.m.
To: Health Watch Group   (59 people in group)
Subject: Ivan—Update
From: Suzanne

Well the results are in. Ivan still has cancer on the tongue and lymph node.

It has been such a mixed up day. First, the speech therapist tells him he is ready to start introducing soft foods and liquids in small portions, the doctor tells him he has gained weight [118.6] and she wants to start 1 can of Ensure® a day and all other issues seem to be clearing up…then the news.

Our next step is next Tuesday with the throat doctor. He indicated he would take a biopsy on the tongue to be sure and then he would discuss our options. So, for now, we wait.

Ivan's spirits are down, as you can imagine. He came home and went to bed and wanted to be alone, so I'm having lunch right now and sending this email. It may seem somber—but it's not the first time we

*have had to lace up the straps and meet this kind of
thing head on. I feel like crying too...but I also don't
want to let my imagination take over and be defeated.*

*Your continued prayers [for strength to accept
God's plan] are greatly appreciated. We know you have
made a difference in our life through this phase...
it's just not over yet...there is more to experience.*

My world was shattered by this latest news. I tried to let people
know how devastated both Ivan and I were, but words could not
describe the scene or the mood in our home. I was crushed to
see my husband retreat inside, curling up on the bed and crying.
How could I fix this when the opponent was so strong, when there
were so many battles to fight?

My world was rocked once again, and I was finding it difficult
to stay positive. I asked others to pray, but I didn't. I thought God
was turning His back on us. I was beginning to feel abandoned
by Him. Although I did not understand why He would do so, I
spent many quiet moments of self-reflection, reliving past events
and trying to figure it out. I had been raised Catholic and had a
strong connection to my faith. I'd attended weekly mass, followed
Catholic practices, and ensured that the girls attended the appro-
priate classes at church. What had I missed?

Guilt was a large component of my faith, and guilt was constant for me. I continued to wonder if there was something we'd
done, or forgotten to do, for which we were being punished. I
believed God rewarded people for their good deeds and punished
others. Clearly, the sequence of events that continued to unfold
was anything but rewarding. We had obviously done something
very wrong.

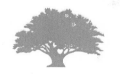

Chapter 30

More News

1/18/2004   *12:41 p.m.*
To: Health Watch Group *(60 people in group)*
Subject: Ivan—Update
From: Suzanne

Just a brief update to let you know the Radiation Oncologist called Friday night to let us know he had reviewed the MRI films and they believe the cancer may have spread to the right vocal cords. This means they will do a biopsy of the area in addition to the base of the tongue to see if their suspicion is correct. He said they are recommending surgery for Ivan's lymph nodes regardless of what they find on the tongue and vocal cords. The biopsy will just tell them how expensive the surgery will be. [Tuesday doctor appointment will hopefully tell us more].

Ivan took the news in stride, stating that he was NOT going to react until they knew the facts. I, on the other hand, have been a mess. I haven't been able to sleep for the last several nights and the news affected me as a result of my lack of sleep.

*Ivan has been cute though. He holds me and says
he understands…*

*Our prayers are that the biopsy will be nothing,
just skin damage from the radiation and then next
step will be simple and easy for Ivan. He has been
excited about eating again and eliminating the feeding line to his vein and I don't blame him. He also
gained another pound! Yeah for him!*

After a five-month roller coaster ride in the medical world, I
felt Ivan wanted to be strong. This had been his style from our
beginning. He saw himself as the man of the house, and this meant
he needed to show courage and strength throughout this illness. I
honestly think that sometimes he appeared to be stronger when I
succumbed to the weight of bad news and cried. As he held me in
his arms and consoled me, I believe it helped him to play the role
of the strong man—the man who was supposed to take care of me.

When Ivan showed such fortitude and strength, I felt challenged to do the same. Ivan had always projected the image of
a strong man before his diagnosis, and I believe that is what he
wanted to be throughout the challenges of his illness. Sometimes,
though, he retreated, cried, or recoiled, and when that happened, I
understood that those behaviors were not his natural response to
challenging situations. Instead, those occasions represented the
frustration and sense of betrayal he felt at times about what was
happening to his body. I was ashamed that I had cried in front of
him and given him cause for concern.

1/21/2004   8:30 a.m.
To: Health Watch Group   (60 people in group)
Subject: Ivan—Update
From: Suzanne

The doctor's exam confirmed that Ivan's lymph node

has cancer remaining, the tongue area remains suspicious, but the vocal cords DO NOT show cancer. He said the vocal cords have been affected by the nerve that is connected in the lymph node area and that's why it showed up as abnormal on the MRI.

The next step is to meet with the surgeon at UCSF for the consultation. He will tell us all of our surgical options and provide more details of the process at that time. The doctor here did indicate that first we would meet with the doctor in SF and then surgery would probably occur a week or so after. We don't know when the appointment for the consultation will be, but it will be on a Thursday [possibly next week or the week after that].

The good news is Ivan now weighs 123 lbs., which means he has gained 10 pounds over the past month. The doctor told us that he now believes Ivan would be able to survive the surgery [whereas he said he did not think this would be the case 2 weeks ago]. He said this was a significant improvement and although they typically would have wanted to perform the surgery right away, in Ivan's case, the catch 22 is that he needs to continue to regain his weight and become stronger in order to have the surgery. So at least the 'waiting' is not 'unproductive' right?

The not-so-good news is that the doctor is concerned about the tumor being 'inoperable'. He said there are several characteristics that make this concerning, but they will only know once they begin the surgery.

Ivan's spirits were down again, as he did not want ANY surgery, but overall he and I talked about the 'good' news in the news.

Thank you for all of your thoughts and prayers.

When Ivan was first diagnosed with cancer, we talked to the physician in California about driving back from Oregon to go to UCSF for treatment. This was discouraged by Ivan. After waiting a couple of weeks to get an appointment, the physician later called with the name of an oncologist in the nearby town of Medford, Oregon. Ivan was grateful for this, as he did not want to travel back to California for treatment or have to deal with the need to spend his nights in a hotel room in San Francisco.

Our early visit to UCSF, immediately after his diagnosis, had been a horrible and frightful experience. The many patients sitting in the waiting room, the disfigured people who had obviously had surgery to remove parts of their face or throat, and the depressing atmosphere of the entire setting made us cringe.

We both worried about the need for us to return to that place after surviving the crisis in ICU and overcoming the many setbacks and the current condition of Ivan's body. That place had been a living nightmare to us, so the thought of adding travel and lonely hotels to the equation was incomprehensible. Medford's cancer center had become the place where we felt safe and cared for. When we learned that we needed to travel back down to California for the expertise of surgical options, we were sickened and worried. Flights were limited and expensive, so driving seemed to be our best option. Unfortunately, the trip had so many twists and turns that we were both exhausted by this latest medical ordeal.

1/21/2004   *12:11 p.m.*
To: Alison
Subject: Ivan —Update
From: Suzanne

The doctor's office called and our appointment is Weds. 1/28 @ 11:00 a.m. We will drive down Tuesday, to stay at mom's [maybe 2 nights] and then drive home Thursday.

1/29/2004　　　　　　　　*6:23 p.m.*
To: Health Watch Group　(60 people in group)
Subject: Ivan—Update
From: Suzanne

For those of you who were not aware, we drove to SF on Tuesday, met with the doctors on Wednesday and drove back to Oregon today [Thursday]. Unfortunately, the trip seemed like a huge punch in the stomach.

After their exam of Ivan they advised us that it is highly unlikely they can do surgery on the lymph node. Ivan's case is being reviewed by the Tumor Board next Wednesday and then the doctor will call with the recommendation, but he told us Ivan's tumor is around the main artery. He said surgery is already bad in that they have to remove/replace part of the artery and that is extremely risky with all of the nerves in the area. He said Ivan's present health situation only makes the already bad situation worse. He is concerned that Ivan could have a heart attack or stroke and end up worse off than when they started. BUT, he did say experts were reviewing the films and data to see if there was a way.

I guess you can appreciate that Ivan and I were both very disappointed and saddened with the news.

The tumor in the lymph node area is growing now again, and the doctor said this is consistent with most cases like this. Although he stated he may not be able to cure Ivan without the surgery, they may propose a new treatment process to try and reduce the tumor and help in his quality of life. He could not give me success ratios because the procedure is new, but we will find out next week if this might be our next option. If this treatment is possible, it is only done in SF so we will need to drive down and stay for a two-week period [which is the amount of time involved with the treatment].

I don't really know what else to say right now. I'm trying to be strong but I'm not doing very good right now. We're praying that everything will be alright, but it's hard to know what that might mean. I'm sure you have questions too, so let me know what I forgot to say and I'll do my best to get back to you.

Love you and thank you for your thoughts and prayers. We're in God's hands.

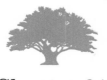

Chapter 31

Faith

In my early childhood days, I was taught that faith was the foundation of life. My parents believed we needed to follow some form of religion in order to strengthen our faith in God, and since my mother was Catholic, my father agreed to allow her to raise the four of us as Catholics.

We followed the practices of Catholicism throughout our childhood, but as my siblings left home and began to raise children of their own, they moved away from the religious practices of the Catholic Church. This was not true for me. I continued to be involved with my Catholic faith.

Ivan's belief in God was strong, and although he had been raised as a Baptist, like my father, he allowed me to raise our children in the Catholic faith as well. I attended mass regularly and made sure both daughters participated in religious classes as they grew up and took the steps necessary to receive the Sacraments of Reconciliation, First Communion, and Confirmation. Faith and God were important to me, and we actively engaged in community events and fundraising activities for the less fortunate. I loved my life in faith and felt valued and fulfilled whenever we spent time giving to others.

Traveling to Oregon to begin our new life as retirees was the beginning of my descent from my faith. I felt betrayed and conflicted about God and the purpose of religion. I did not attend mass during Ivan's eight-month ordeal. During that entire time, I denied my faith and believed that God had forsaken me—and that He had forsaken Ivan as well. I felt my religious life had been a sham and whatever I had done to deserve the hand we'd been dealt was overwhelming to me. I spoke of God to others, but I felt empty. I had transferred my feelings of inadequacy to my faith in God and did not feel worthy of His love, let alone anyone else's. Pity was my internal partner.

Throughout Ivan's illness, I was overwhelmed with sorrow. I wrote, "We're in God's hands," but I didn't believe it. I felt God had let our dreams and prayers slip through His fingers. He wasn't with us, holding us close or keeping us safe. We were alone and forsaken, and my disappointment was profound and ran deep. Each day, I struggled to not cry in front of Ivan. I'm sure he knew I was in an internal battle. It was becoming impossible to imagine hope. There seemed to be no light at the end of this horrific tunnel, and no relief from the medical problems. We were caught in a current of "one thing after another" taking us further downstream. I was becoming weary, and it was all I could do to just get through the day.

What I didn't tell everyone was the fact that the doctor's message contained more bad news. I couldn't find it in my heart to tell people what was really going on. This would acknowledge how powerful cancer had become and that it seemed to be winning the battle. I couldn't tell them that, but Alison did.

1/30/2004   *9:11 a.m.*
To: Health Watch Grou   *(60 people in group) p*
Subject: Ivan—Update
From: Alison

Here is the latest update…not good news. We are hanging in there the best we can but it's pretty tough for us right now.

What mom left out of the email is that last night they got a call from the Oncologist in Oregon. Dad's blood work has showed that there is something wrong with his liver. This was the only organ that was doing ok. Mom and dad are at the hospital right now where they are doing a test of dad's liver. We find out the results of the test today at 3:00 p.m. Needless to say we are all sad, scared and frustrated…and mom is becoming more and more fearful of what may come our way…as we all are.

Alison's message was clear. She was fearful that Ivan might die, and yet she struggled to state that openly to me. She had been our light and hope through her constant calling and presence. Her strength and joyful demeanor had helped me to maintain a positive attitude. She was beginning to see the situation differently, and this scared her. It frightened me even more.

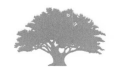

Chapter 32

Denied

2/06/2004   2:25 p.m.
To: Health Watch Group   (60 people in group)
Subject Ivan—Update
From: Suzanne

The doctor has confirmed that the Tumor Board did not approve any surgery to remove the cancer. They did however approve Ivan for the Hyperthermal Radiation treatment, which will help his quality of life [and could create a remission…who knows].

We are scheduled to drive down to the Bay Area on 2/12 and stay with my mom in Pleasanton. Our first appointment will be Friday the 13th. We don't have very much information about the treatment itself, except that it will last 2 weeks. [It's a fairly new treatment with the use of microwaves.]

Since I wrote last, Ivan has had a problem with his gallbladder and they are recommending removal, but we believe it can wait until we complete the new treatment program.

I will try to write before we leave [if there is further information] but I don't believe I will be able to write once we are in the Bay Area.

Thank you all for your continued support and I ask that you continue to pray for Ivan! You have been so instrumental in his recovery so far that we are blessed to have you as friends!

While we managed the news from the tumor board, the oncologist discovered that the earlier test on the liver appeared to indicate that Ivan's gallbladder was involved. She feared that the cancer had traveled to other organs, specifically to the gallbladder. I didn't share her suspicion with the Health Watch Group. It felt like another acknowledgment of cancer's tenacity, and I couldn't get myself to accept this.

2/18/2004   9:40 a.m.
To: Health Watch Group   (60 people in group)
Subject: Ivan—Update
From: Suzanne

When we went to the doctor on Friday at UCSF, we were surprised and disappointed to have the doctor tell us that she did not think Ivan was a candidate for the Hyperthermal treatment. She agreed to review the file, films and talk to other doctors, so we were sent home and waited until Tuesday to get a call from her.

Yesterday she called and asked that we drive to the city right away to meet with another specialist in this field. We did—and he told us he thought he could do the treatment, despite the complexity of the area. They will insert needle-like rods in the area around the lymph nodes and heat the area with these rods.

The rods will remain in the neck until the treatment is complete. Friday we will tentatively set up to have the pretreatment process [rods inserted, etc.] and Monday we should begin the 5-day treatment. Beyond this, we don't have any other information about the process, timing, etc.

We will stay at my mom's until 2/28, when we will return to Oregon. As usual, please understand Ivan or I may not always be able to talk or meet, but we will do our best.

To try to articulate the feeling of the up-and-down emotions during this period was extremely difficult. Each time we struggled to stand and be strong, we were knocked down by more health issues. Ivan was losing physical weight, like a boxer in a never-ending fight, and I was losing "emotional weight." My reserves were depleted, and I felt weak. This emotional up and down took its toll on me, and I found that I had to go numb in order to go on. I knew I could not physically handle any more distressing news about Ivan's health. I needed to tune it out or I would become useless in my caregiver role. I did not focus on what was being said or what I was doing; I was just performing the required functions, completely disconnected from the severity of Ivan's situation or how I felt.

If I connected to the severity of his health issues, and the overwhelming number of things I needed to manage, I felt I would crumble, and the cancer would win. Unconsciously, I decided not to listen to the potential ramifications of the information the doctors stated. It seemed as if my brain took over, allowing me to continue physically with my caregiver duties, as my heart retreated somewhere into the recesses of my gut. This was a safe place for it, so I didn't have to feel the heavy gloom of each day.

With my heart safely tucked away, I could smile, take care of my husband, and remain strong in my convictions that it would all work out in the end. This approach was familiar to me—I'd been trained early in life to bury my emotions. By listening to my brain and thinking through everything I needed to do, I did not have to listen to my heart and show my vulnerability. I could keep strong. I could feel in control, although control was terribly elusive during this time.

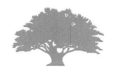

Chapter 33

Heart Treatment

2/21/2004   *8:52 a.m.*
To: Health Watch Group   *(60 people in group)*
Subject: Ivan—Update
From: Suzanne

We met with the doctor again on Friday and after a full review they have decided NOT to do the treatment.

They told us that the symptoms are the same right now between the old tumor reacting to the radiation and dying off and a NEW growth that is spreading. He said that Ivan had the maximum radiation and therefore more rays [which is included in the Hyperthermal] could create holes in his jugular vein and kill him. We were told to go back home, have a scan in about 3 weeks and then if the tumor is viewed as growing, they will discuss our 'options'.

We're not sad...too much. I have to tell you that in the car on our way back to my mom's house from SF it was silent...and then Ivan said he "had this figured out". He said, "someone out there is not doing their job and praying, that's all." We both burst out laughing...so I wanted to tell you, so you know we are okay.

We believe God had us here...not for the treatment of the tumor, but for the treatment of our heart. To see friends and family has been great and therapeutic for both of us. So we will go back to Oregon and wait for God's next plan. And who knows...maybe the cancer is dying off and the sadness will end soon. Each doctor has their own opinion of the situation, so why can't we have ours too.

My mom's birthday is on the 24th, so we leave after that and drive back to Oregon.

Ivan had been raised a Baptist during his childhood in Arkansas, but he did not continue to practice his faith once he left home. He was spiritual but not religious. He often read the Bible at night before retiring to bed and joined a Bible reading group a few years before we retired. Ivan believed there was a higher power, and after he became a recovering alcoholic, that belief became even stronger. He believed his faith in God helped him stay clean and sober. He often referred to the importance of trusting in God and letting go of trying to control life. The slogan, "Let go and let God," became a common phrase he used whenever troubles occurred for anyone he knew. However, since learning of his illness, if he prayed or let go, it was not apparent.

Ivan had also always stated, "God has a plan, and He's on time." He said it to remind us that attempts to worry or control any outcome were futile, if not comical. Ivan held firmly to the belief that there was a plan for everything and acceptance of that plan was our role in life. But as he seemed to retreat inside more and more, I wondered if he was struggling to trust in God after all. He never picked up the Bible anymore. I thought he was finding it difficult to understand how his illness was part of a plan he could accept. We never spoke of his faith while he was ill. Although he sometimes showed anger toward his deteriorating body, most of the time he quietly moved through the day without showing extreme emotions or expressing his thoughts and feelings. At least this is what I thought because it was how I was managing my own faith.

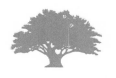

Chapter 34

Pneumonia

3/02/2004   5:00 p.m.
To: Health Watch Group   (60 people in group)
Subject: Ivan—Update
From: Suzanne

Last Tuesday [2/24] we drove direct from my mother's home in California back to Ivan's doctor's office. He had a high fever the day before and felt sick most of the day, so I was concerned about his lungs.

He was diagnosed with pneumonia and instead of being admitted to the hospital, we traveled to the infusion center each day for 7 days for the IV drip antibiotic. Today, we were told the pneumonia is gone! Yeah...

Next week he will have the tests he needs to see if the cancer is growing or not. He will have a CT scan, PET and an MRI.

We are now working on giving him more water and liquid in his stomach tube. He is still on the TPN through the vein, so our goal is to ramp up on tube feedings, ramp down on TPN and eventually introduce food and drink orally. This may take months, but we are going to start the transition again [our last try failed and caused him to get sick and become impacted, so we had to stop].

He weighs 129 and so many people thought he looked great, as a result of his weight...and he does!

Thanks for your emails asking for updates. I never know when enough is enough, so I hold off writing some of the time.

I struggled to send any communication to people after February 24. The days and weeks following that date were spent managing Ivan's pneumonia. I had called the doctor from my mom's home in California once I realized he was looking sickly. As soon as I took his temperature, I called the oncologist and spoke directly with her on the phone. She instructed me to get back to Oregon as soon as possible and drive directly to the hospital. She said they would have a bed waiting for him.

The drive took six hours, and Ivan moaned and winced every time I hit a bump in the road. His was nauseated and in pain. I drove as fast as I could, wincing internally at the pain of our situation. This illness was beating both of us down. I did not want to go back to the hospital. I didn't want to go back to the regimen of sleepless nights and days full of uncertainties, of ups and downs, due to Ivan's changing condition. I adjusted to each situation as it occurred, but I wanted the constant health issues to stop.

I was tired and wanted this roller coaster ride to be over. I needed Ivan to be well. I knew he needed to go back to the hospital. His health demanded it. But I was conflicted between the guilt of worrying about my own feelings, his current health crisis, and my fear of what lay ahead back in Medford.

When we returned to Medford, Ivan spent the first few days in the hospital, and his pneumonia improved. Since his hospitalization was brief, I didn't bother to tell people about it.

The fact that we were able to manage the condition outside of the hospital turned out to be both a blessing and a curse—the blessing to be home and able to take care of the pets and other chores, but the curse of added travel back and forth from the infusion center. After writing this email, Ivan again became very ill. His temperature spiked, and his vomit was black with blood from the internal issues that were going on. I did not write to tell people about this latest setback. I believed this was just another episode with his lungs and that things would improve again, as they always had. He was admitted back into the hospital on March 3. They found he was impacted once again, and the issues of the gallbladder and intestinal tract being invaded by the cancer remained a concern for the oncologist.

He stayed in the hospital for five days, until March 8, when the oncologist asked me to step out of his hospital room and sit down with her in a nearby office.

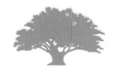

Chapter 35

Robbed

In the small office that was situated a few doors down from Ivan's room, the physician had tears in her eyes as she spoke of Ivan's choices. He could stay at the hospital or return home with hospice. She told me that they felt Ivan had about five days left to live. She talked about the many health issues they had found and how they believed the cancer had manifested in almost all of his organs.

I sat there, stunned. I did not break into tears. I was shocked by her words. How could this be? We had come so far. We had been through so much. I just stared at her. I had not comprehended or believed the situation was this bad. I had been so busy fighting off the sharks that I hadn't grasped the depth of his illness. What was she saying? I thought each step we'd taken was moving Ivan toward getting better, but it seemed I had become immune to the reality of the events that had transpired. After she explained the situation to me, we entered the hospital room to talk to Ivan.

As the oncologist spoke to Ivan and held his hand, she explained his choices. She did not tell him about all the health issues they had found that she had conveyed to me, but she stated clearly to him that they would arrange hospice if he elected to go home.

Ivan elected to go home and seemed pleased. He only spoke about the fact that he could go back home and get well there—better than in the hospital. He didn't seem to realize what was being explained to him—that he would not survive this illness. He acted like he was going home to get stronger, and this was difficult for me to listen to and watch. I smiled as he looked at me and spoke as if we were going to beat this illness. He was on strong pain medicine, and I thought this was why he did not seem to connect with her words.

I felt empty as I stood there, listening to the doctor talk to Ivan. We were not going to spend countless days by the river fishing together. We were not going to spend romantic moments dining in new places. There would be no shared joys of birthdays or holidays or new grandchildren yet to be born. Cancer had stolen our future, our possibilities. Cancer had robbed us of our retirement, our happiness. I was still in shock, trying to comprehend the gravity of the words she was speaking, but deep inside, I knew that everything had changed. I stared at Ivan and thought of Christmas Day, lying on the bed crying in each other's arms, believing that next Christmas would be better. We would not have another Christmas together. Ivan would not get better. This was it.

3/09/2004   *9:33 a.m.*
To: Health Watch Group   (60 people in group)
Subject: Ivan—Update
From: Suzanne

I don't know how to start this email except to say we have some sad news.

We were informed yesterday that Ivan's tumor is growing rapidly. They also found he has infections or tumors in his gallbladder, spleen and lungs. He had been taken off TPN and is at home now, with hospice expected to arrive today. Our goal is pain management to keep him comfortable.

His character is to remain strong and determined, and so are we.

We thank you for your prayers and thoughts during these difficult days.

This was not everything Ivan's doctor had shared with me. They found cancer in his gallbladder, lungs, and spleen. They also found cancer in his liver, urinary tract, and intestines, as well as in the original lymph node and his throat. He still had difficulty swallowing, his increased bedsores exposed his tail bone, and he was in pain throughout his entire body.

We still needed to watch his blood pressure, for fear of stroke and skin sensitivity, due to the medicines. His oncologist worried that his condition would be too much for me to manage at home and hoped he would select to stay in the hospital, where the staff could care for his many challenging issues.

The gravity of the information was numbing. I tried to listen as she spoke of him remaining in the hospital, but I wasn't really hearing her. In my mind, I kept replaying over and over the movie of her first few words, "We have found cancer throughout Ivan's body."

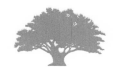

Chapter 36

The Gift

We had a hospital bed delivered to the house, and I quickly set up all the supplies I again would need to care for Ivan. Before bringing Ivan home, I stopped by several medical supplies stores, as I had done once before.

His bedsores had worsened again from the stay in the hospital, and his tailbone protruded, exposing the slender white bone underneath. The special care required to tend to this open wound was difficult to perform without causing significant pain to Ivan. I had to delicately clean the area with wound care medicine and place a wide gauze bandage over the area. The bandage material and the tape I used were lightweight, due to the sensitivity of his skin. If the tape was too tight against the thin, flaky skin, his skin would attach to the bandage material and peel off with the tape.

When the hospice nurse arrived the day after Ivan came home, she walked through the health issues I needed to manage and helped me plan his daily care: pills every two hours (which needed to be crushed and administered through the stomach tube), replacement of the battery for his clavicle vein med-pack (which dispensed continual morphine), and diapers and bandage replacements every couple of hours, along with hourly thermometer readings, blood pressure readings, and mouth swabbing. We didn't need to feed Ivan since his system could no longer process food, but because he could not swallow, the regular application of water-soaked swabs was critical. I also had sheepskin pads for his bedsores and absorbent pads for unexpected incontinence.

I was going through each of the motions with purpose and with as much energy as I could muster. This was the only way for me to stave off what I knew was coming. My role had drastically changed from helping the nurses at the hospital to becoming his final nurse at home. I had been his nurse at home before, but this time it was more intense. Ivan's extended life and comfort were in my hands. Each task I needed to perform was essential to ensure his relief from pain. I did not spend time thinking about my misery, discomfort, or fears. I needed to pay attention to the details of his care. I had a new reason for existing, and it consumed me.

3/23/2004 *7:25 p.m.*
To: Health Watch Group (60 people in group)
Subject: Ivan—Update
From: Suzanne

I realized after talking with my family that most of you are anxious to hear how things are going, so I'll try to update you while keeping it brief.

When we came home from the hospital, hospice thought Ivan had about a week to live. That was 15 days ago. He is off feeding, weighs 100 pounds and is resting comfortably most of the time, but does not speak anymore.

They believe his liver is failing, among other issues and so I stay by his side as much as possible.

Although the kids have gone, my mom is here and has helped a lot with the cooking, cleaning and watching Ivan while I rest at times in the day. He is restless when he is awake, which is about every two hours.

What can I say? Except that we pray every day for Ivan to be at peace physically and mentally. Although the situation is very sad, I think about the nurse's comment. She said a person's character does not change in death from that which it was in life—therefore, it is no surprise that Ivan is strong, a fighter, and such a proud man. I believe this is the gift he is showing me, and I will always remember this about him...not the physical condition that is before me.

Although a celebration will occur in the Bay Area in the future, we will let you know in due time. Until then, bless you all for giving us these days and for your part in the incredible journey with us.

May God hold you in His arms, as He holds Ivan.

When Ivan first arrived home on March 9, he remained strong and talked about returning to work to rebuild some of the loss of income we were experiencing. Both of our daughters came to see their father a few days after he arrived home, and during their stay, he spoke of having them start a new company together with the two of us, so we could rebuild and restore our income quicker. As he spoke, it seemed as if he was in denial. When we sat together one evening, he told me he wanted to talk to the doctor again to find out what was next. I was shocked. He did not seem to grasp the gravity of his fate.

When I reminded him that we had been sent home because there was nothing more they could do for us, he became angry and insisted that he speak to the doctor. He accused me of being dramatic and felt a call with the physician would clarify the situation. Although it was the oncologist who had informed Ivan of his condition and the need for hospice, Ivan insisted that he talk to the radiologist since he believed further treatment was possible. I arranged for a call with the radiologist, and both of our daughters listened in on the other telephone extensions.

The doctor told Ivan he only had days to live, and there was nothing more that could be done. There was silence on the line for several minutes, and then Ivan thanked him for his time. The doctor kept apologizing to Ivan, saying he was "sorry, so sorry," but Ivan did not respond. He hung up.

This conversation changed Ivan. He became somber once again and did not speak after the call. The girls cried as they spoke to me about the call and Ivan's lack of acknowledgment of his actual condition. The remaining couple of days for the girls were dismal around the house. He did not talk to them about his dying, nor did he discuss his health at all. When they left to return home, they kissed Ivan, and he told them goodbye. But as the days came and went after their departure, Ivan never spoke to me again.

Each day the hospice nurse visited the house to check on Ivan and make sure I was administering the pain medicine, as well as properly treating his open wound. It had been sixteen days since the doctor told me Ivan had five days left to live, so one day the nurse asked me, "What's keeping this man alive? Is there someone he is waiting to see?" I told her no, that there was nothing, but she insisted that something was keeping him alive, and only time would tell us what it was. She told me about other cases where once a family arrived or the individual received a call they had been waiting for, they passed away quietly. Again, I told her there was no one and nothing.

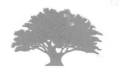

Chapter 37

The Vision

O n March 24, as I walked into the bedroom to administer his treatment, Ivan reached out his hand and smiled, greeting me as if I were a long-lost friend, and said, "Great to see you!" in his soft, whispering tone. This was the first time he had spoken to me since the call with the radiologist. I felt a rush of love come over me, believing he had forgiven me for the wrong decisions I had made, forgiven me for the many times I had administered the painful treatment for his open bedsores, forgiven me for changing his diaper or washing his face as if he were an infant, forgiven me for being the person who had made him face his fate. My husband was reaching out his hand to me, and I felt incredibly loved.

I smiled and walked toward him, extending my hand to embrace his. As I took each step closer, the man before me changed, and the scene I was watching felt as if it were in slow motion.

Left foot forward: his hand extended toward me, and his eyes sparkled.

Right foot forward: his head shook slightly, as if trying to clear his vision.

Left foot forward: his eyes widened slightly to take in the person he was seeing—me.

Right foot forward: his facial expression changed to disgust.

As I grasped his hand, he abruptly pulled his hand away and turned his head to the side. He did not look at me. Apparently, he'd thought I was someone else. Possibly the medicine had caused him to hallucinate, or a dream or vision led him to believe he was seeing someone else, but whatever he'd seen, the damage was done. I was crushed. My husband had not been happy to see *me*; he had not forgiven me. The words he spoke would be his last. Sadly, I knew they had not been meant for me.

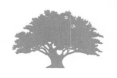

Chapter 38

Time

3/25/2004   *4:43 p.m.*
To: Health Watch Group   (60 people in group)
Subject: Ivan—Update
From: Alison

Hello everyone,

I want you all to know that Ivan's condition has changed again...the hospice nurse came out today and told mom he would probably pass this afternoon or tonight. He is not moving or talking anymore, and his breaths are about 30-35 seconds apart. Therefore, I wanted all of you to know that in the event of his death, I will be taking off to Oregon, which could mean tomorrow. Unfortunately, my cell phone reception is horrible at mom's house but I have learned how to check my messages on it so I will be checking them. You can also email me.

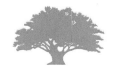

Chapter 39

The Other Women

How do I begin to talk to my two daughters about the impending death of their father? This was something I had not considered or accepted during the past several months. I had been in denial about the magnitude of his illness, and I could not find it in myself to speak to the girls about this inevitable outcome.

I talked to Alison daily, and sometimes more than twice a day. She was living the horrific days with me, and we spoke about Ivan's discomfort or pain, but we never spoke the word "death" out loud. She was strong, caring, and entrenched in the sadness of losing Ivan, so I'm sure she must have been contemplating his fate.

Sara was expecting but had been placed on restrictions due to the delicacy of her pregnancy. She had been showing signs of a possible miscarriage, and her doctor felt the stress of her father's illness was affecting her. When I talked to her, I tried not to share too much because I worried about her health. There was no way I would talk to her about Ivan dying. While I was able to hug Alison in person whenever she came to the house, I could only hug Sara virtually through the phone. We could not have the physical connection we both desperately needed.

I loved both of my girls dearly and watched them emerge as grown women through this sad experience. I was proud of the women both of my children had become, but still, I was not prepared to talk to them about the death of their father. I could not and did not. This was too sad for me, and I did not have the emotional strength.

Although I couldn't speak to them about the reality of what was happening to our family, the days of talking to them about wishful thinking and dreaming of fun moments again with Ivan in our future were gone. This tore my heart apart—watching him dying and not being able to talk to either of them about it or the future of our family without their father. As I reflect on them now, I realize how lonely this time must have felt for them too. Cancer had destroyed their father and left their emotions abandoned by, and isolated from me, in its wake.

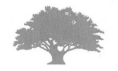

Chapter 40

Uplifting Energy

In the early morning of March 26, I had gone to the kitchen, some twenty yards away, to get Ivan's medicine. When I returned, he was not in his hospital bed. My eyes darted frantically and landed on the small figure of a man sitting in the chair beside the bed. The guardrails of the hospital bed were still up and everything else seemed normal, except Ivan was desperately trying to hold himself upright in the chair. I quickly raced to his side to catch him from falling.

My heart was pounding and my arms shook as I struggled to get him back into the bed. He only weighed between eighty and ninety pounds, but it was still difficult to lift him. I started to panic as I lowered the side rail and tried to push him up onto the bed. This took all the energy I had, but I managed.

Once in bed, he rolled onto his side, and I covered him with the sheet. He returned to the deep sleep he had been in for the last few days. I stared at the small figure in the bed and stood there perplexed, wondering how he'd been able to lift himself over the guardrails and into the chair in the short amount of time it took for me to walk from the bedroom to the kitchen and back again; how had he done it?

I recalled the time my father had been in the hospital, dying of cancer, and the nurse told us a story about how my father had scared her when she went in to check on him. Apparently, he was sitting up in a chair beside the hospital bed, despite his frail condition and the bedside guardrails that were up. It was the night before my father died. I wondered if Ivan was in his final hours too.

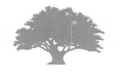

Chapter 41

3.26
More than Numbers

Alison drove up from California that Friday, March 26, as she had done every weekend for the past several weeks. She was a great comfort and support to me as the days progressed. My sister Lynn also decided to join us, and after a snowy drive from the Bay Area to Oregon, she sat with my mom in the living room and watched TV as I stayed with Ivan in the bedroom.

Around 2:00 p.m., the phone rang. It was Sara, calling from San Diego. She told me they had just come from the doctor's office and found out they were having a baby boy. They had waited to tell us that they'd planned to learn the sex of the baby, hoping they would find out if she was carrying a boy. She said that since the baby was indeed a boy, they wanted to give him the middle name of "Ivan."

Sara asked if she could tell her father herself about their news and their plan to give the baby Ivan's name. I gently held the phone to Ivan's ear and told Sara to talk. Ivan did not open his eyes as she told him the news about his namesake.

This was a happy but unexpected call. The words of the hospice nurse rang in my head. (The hospice nurse would later insist that this was the call Ivan had been waiting to receive before he could die peacefully—giving this gift to Sara of being alive to hear her news.)

Around 3:15 p.m., I decided to lay down on the bed in our room (which was positioned next to Ivan's hospital bed). As I lay there on my back, staring at the ceiling, I listened to the rhythm of Ivan's breathing. It was slow and methodical and had a calming feel to it. In out, in..............out, in.................out, silence.

I sat up, looked at Ivan's chest, and waited for the movement of his body to take a breath in. It did not come. I glanced at the clock. It was 3:26 p.m. *Is he dead?*

I moved from my bed, stood beside his hospital bed, and continued to watch his body. The rhythm had stopped. He was no longer breathing. He was gone. At 3:26 p.m., on March 26, he had departed. Tears flowed from my eyes as I acknowledged that he was no longer with us. I slowly and carefully slipped onto his bed to lay beside his frail body. I rested my head on his shoulder and quietly sobbed. Cancer had taken my love. Cancer had drained the energy from my husband's arms, which were unable to hold me as I wept.

I knew I needed to get up from beside him and tell my daughter the news, but I lay there for several minutes, wishing he would move—wishing he would breathe so we could continue our fight. His skin was cold to the touch, and I knew our life together had ended. I kissed him on his lips, for what was to be the last time.

An enormous sense of inadequacy came over me—a sense of loss, a sense of desolation, a sense of exhaustion, and an incredible sense of failure. I had failed to save my love. Of all the strength and courage I had found in my life to master other situations and other life challenges, I had not succeeded at the most important challenge of all. I felt incredibly empty and alone at that moment.

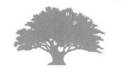

Chapter 42

Peace

After several minutes, I got up, opened the bedroom door, and informed Alison, my sister, and my mom that Ivan had passed away. Alison ran into my arms and openly wept, while my sister and mom entered the bedroom to verify that Ivan had departed.

3/26/2004   *6:13 p.m.*
To: Health Watch Group   (60 people in group)
Subject: Ivan—Update
From: Suzanne

This afternoon our prayers for Ivan to be at peace were heard.

Ivan ended his fight with cancer and joined God at 3:26 p.m.

We will have a private service at our home on Sunday and then travel to the Bay Area for a celebration on Thursday, April 1.

Moving Forward...
Walking Backward

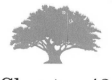

Chapter 43

Strength

For several months, I struggled to accept the loss of my husband. My grief counselor told me that the loss of Ivan, who had been my business partner as well as my companion of twenty-five years, would take five to seven years for me to recover from. I dismissed this idea. I was stronger than that.

I thought it would only take three months or so to regain myself and move forward. After all, I was a strong, positive person, and the thought of grieving for such a long period of time made me feel weak. People expected me to grieve; they expected me to act a certain way. But after a "reasonable period of time" they expected me to be strong and move forward with my life, right? Or is that what I expected of myself?

I believed I needed to be strong, like my mother had been when my father passed away. She cried and was miserable for a while, but after a couple of months, she seemed to regain her strength and assumed the role of matriarch for our family. I wasn't sure I could do that, but I needed to pretend I could—for the sake of my daughters, if for no one else.

Each day I woke up, washed my face, brushed my teeth, dressed, and pasted the smile on my face that sat beside the mirror. I had placed this fake smile on my face since the beginning of Ivan's illness, so it was easy to continue to do this. I would not let cancer ruin my life. It would not conquer me too.

As I moved through the day, my resistance to depression became more and more difficult to maintain. My sleep pattern remained the same, as when I had cared for Ivan. I woke up every two hours and remained awake for two to three hours at a time. The lack of sleep began to undermine my ability to fight depression.

On some days, I could not get out of bed. I was tired, heartbroken, and alone—alone in the large home in the country that we had only moved into eight months earlier. I felt sorry for myself. I had lost my purpose for living. True, I had two lovely daughters, but I began to feel that they were grown, married, and had their own lives to live. I felt cancer had taken away my reason for living. My relationship with Ivan meant everything, and yet cancer had killed that when it killed him. I found little joy in pretending I could succeed at anything else in life. I hated the disease and the terrible sadness it left in its wake. Cancer had won and taken my love, and I wanted to go too. I was of no value to anyone else.

After twenty-five years of being with someone, I realized that my life had become "the two of us," however independent I had been in our marriage. I found it hard to shift from what we wanted to what I wanted. I had not imagined that I would be on my own. I had been confident that we would beat cancer, so it seemed ludicrous that I was facing life alone. That feeling created guilt for thinking I could do whatever I wanted or that I could be happy after the loss of Ivan. I felt angry that Ivan got to die, but I was left to live on…alone. I had always envisioned our lives together, and I even thought we would die together. I never considered my life without him.

I held on to the anger toward Ivan and repeatedly felt sorry for myself. Ivan had always been the person to focus on our financial goals; he had always taken care of the ambitions and visions for our future. I was responsible for the day-to-day functions, the operations, so to speak—bills, household maintenance, our schedule, etc. *Why did I have to do it all now? Why me?*

We had planned our retirement, and our financial situation was perfect. We never planned on the series of events that occurred prior to Ivan's illness: having to take legal action against the new owner of our former company to fight for the money they owed us; selling our home in California at a greatly reduced amount, due to the unexpected downturn in the housing market; or managing unanticipated medical expenses associated with Ivan's conditions. After Ivan's death, other income sources also ceased, such as his social security and one of his retirement plans. (Neither of us realized that I would not be eligible for his social security because I was not sixty years old or the fact that one of his retirement plans did not have a survivor benefit.) The reality of my new financial circumstances was unexpected and worrisome. I was left to figure out a new financial path for myself—to determine what actions I needed to take to ensure that I would be financially secure. Having to make these determinations was new to me and created another area of my life that made me feel sorry for myself.

The burdens of the finances, as well as the maintenance of our large house and acreage, turned into perfect excuses for my disengagement from my family and friends. I was a martyr on the inside who smiled on the outside. I shared my anger toward Ivan with my counselor but not with my friends. After all, I felt this was inappropriate and disrespectful toward Ivan. But that didn't stop the internal destruction that was occurring as a result of these feelings. The more I dwelled on my burdens, my anger, and my fear of the future, the more depression took root.

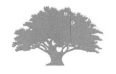

Chapter 44

Over the Shoulder

A couple of months after Ivan passed away, my physician referred me to Marsha, a grief counselor, and I met with her once a week for three years. Marsha prescribed medication to help me sleep and to alter my depression, but I still struggled to find reasons to get up in the morning.

As I worked around the house, fixing and repairing things, I thought of Ivan. He had been a handyman, and I had learned a lot from him. I decided to apply what I'd learned to take charge of things the way Ivan would have. I lay in bed at night, trying to think of everything I could do to keep Ivan's memory alive within myself and in my daily life—to continue my sense of "we" forever.

I began to make financial decisions, household decisions, and even relationship decisions that were based on what Ivan would want to see happen. Everything I did was based on looking back—looking over my shoulder at what once was and how I could regain it again if I were smart. I would show Ivan that I was capable of living how he would have wanted us to.

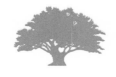

Chapter 45

Weight

A round nine months after losing Ivan, I looked in the mirror and was sickened by what I saw. I had gained forty pounds during the time I cared for Ivan, which only added to my disgust with myself. I was still carrying the weight, which served as another proof point that I was failing to manage my life. The truth is that there had been no time to exercise or prepare healthy meals. My role as caregiver was time-consuming and engulfed my life. Since Ivan's death, I hadn't done much to improve my self-care. Depression had become my new master.

I started putting money into the care, maintenance, and transformation of the house and the grounds. I began to physically work around the six and a half acres. I learned how to operate an old 750 stick shift John Deere tractor, along with the brush hog attachment on the back. It was difficult at first to gain confidence in my ability to work the machine, but I slowly mastered cutting the long field grass in the pasture with the brush hog and moving dirt and other debris with the front-loader bucket. For a girl who had never changed the oil in a car, I totally restored this tractor and was a frequent visitor to the John Deere dealer for parts.

I woke up early and worked around the property from seven in the morning until seven in the evening each day. I came into the house for water or a snack, but otherwise, my day was filled with repairing sprinkler heads, replacing landscape lighting bulbs, trimming bushes, weeding, or laying rock pathways. The grounds began to transform, and so did I. I loved this work. It required me to focus on what I was doing and not on my sorrow. I was exhausted at the end of each day, and although I still had difficulty sleeping, come morning, I had enough energy again for the heavy landscape work.

Before I started my work around the property, Sara had come out to visit and stayed for a few weeks with Jarrod Ivan, my new grandson. When she saw how much weight I had gained after Ivan's passing, she was shocked. She asked me what the heck I was doing to myself and immediately committed to a program to help me lose weight. She bought the book *The South Beach Diet* and began figuring out a diet regimen for me. We purchased an elliptical and set up a workout room in the screened-in porch on the second floor. We began to run every morning to and from the mailbox before we ate our breakfast. This was a morning mile run. She kicked my butt, and I loved that she cared so much about helping me regain my life.

After Sara left, I also began to paint both the inside and outside of the house. The two-story home had high-pitched ceilings, and I assembled two layers of scaffolding, in order to reach the top of the walls in some of the rooms. This was difficult to do on my own, and I broke into tears on more than one occasion when I found the equipment too heavy for me to assemble. Each time, after sitting on the floor of the room and having a good cry, I picked myself up and tried again until I found a way to set up the scaffolding. I felt proud of my accomplishments, and I knew Ivan would have been proud too. After all, I was tackling things I had never done before, using tools and equipment I never imagined I could manage.

Time passed, and I was successfully completing projects. I transformed the home from its earlier worn-and-tired appearance to a new-and-healthy look. My appearance was transforming too. I lost the forty pounds, as well as five additional pounds I had gained before I started the diet Sara prescribed. I was becoming lean and fit.

The work around the home and the property took me almost twelve months to complete. As I finished each project in the house or around the property, I stood and admired my work. But the feeling of satisfaction was always overridden by an overwhelming feeling of emptiness. I could not seem to shake this feeling no matter how hard I worked, no matter how many projects I completed, and no matter how busy I kept myself. The outcome was always the same—emptiness. I knew Ivan would have approved of my accomplishments. I knew he would have been proud of me. So why did I still feel so empty? I asked myself this repeatedly, but the only answer that vibrated in my mind was the fact that I was alone, regardless of what I accomplished.

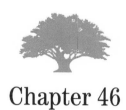

Chapter 46

Finances

In the early months after Ivan's passing, I charted our assets. I created a balance sheet, which helped me understand exactly how much I had left in our accounts. I knew I would need to return to work. The numbers told me that. But I was not ready to go back to the former type of work I'd done—not without Ivan. I felt inadequate and incapable of performing those functions without him by my side.

I had previously been referred to as a workaholic by my friends and employees because I spent long hours at my job. Affectionately, of course, but the fact was I loved my work and was extremely passionate about the results I achieved in the insurance industry. I was a perfectionist and a success-driven person. The thought of trying to recapture this level of energy, especially without Ivan being a part of my efforts, was simply unimaginable to me.

Before I started working on the property around June 2004, I was approached by a dear friend in New York, who asked me to come to work for him. The job would be similar to what Ivan and I had done before we retired. I agreed to come on board, and after about three months of grieving, I began working from home and traveling to New York on business. The smile I took off the shelf each morning was getting heavier and more difficult to manage, but I kept going anyway. I was sinking into a hole of depression, fueled by my feelings of inadequacy and failure, but I didn't realize it at the time. I was focused on doing a great job, pretending to be happy, and building back my financial stability.

I mentally criticized everything I did on the job, finding fault with the littlest things about myself. My friend wanted me to assume more and more responsibility. He felt he was helping me by offering me the opportunity to work. However, I was aware that he also needed to justify my position to his other business partners. He had extended himself by bringing me into the company, and this burden weighed heavily on me. One morning, I woke up and realized I couldn't do it anymore. I could not continue the charade of being excited about working again.

After just three months of work, I was losing my desire to live. During a session with my grief counselor, she identified the depth of my pain and suffering. At first, Marsha threatened to place me in a hospital, where they could monitor me and help me manage my depression. This made me mad. I felt that no one could understand the pain I was going through, and only I had the right to determine what I wanted and needed. She threatened to admit me to the hospital unless I promised not to hurt myself and to follow her advice—to stop working, begin medication, and increase my counseling sessions to uncover some of the emotions I had been blocking. Reluctantly, I agreed. I did not want to be admitted to the hospital, but I was afraid of the suicidal thoughts I'd been dealing with.

When I called my friend to tell him of my decision to stop work, he was furious. He had gone out of his way to help me and was angry that I had not given him more respect or appreciation for his efforts. He yelled at me and called me a "ditcher." When it was clear that I was not going to change my mind, he hung up on me. We did not speak again for several months, but the damage to our relationship was permanent.

Although I did what was necessary to help myself, I could not shake the feeling that once again I'd messed up. Although unintentional, I had let down a good friend. My self-recrimination for being a "ditcher" joined the pile of proof points of my inadequacy, which sent me into deeper despair.

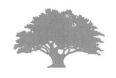

Chapter 47

Work

I avoided the opportunity to return to the workforce for two years following Ivan's death. Around May 2006, I began to work as a consultant for a former client. I was worried about my financial well-being, and this work was neither difficult nor demanding. It allowed me to create an income source. Since a lot of my assets were being spent on replacement vehicles, home improvements, and travel to family, I needed to focus my attention on employment and working again in the industry where I had thirty-two years of experience.

Although the client wanted to hire me as one of their senior executives, I declined their overtures. I was not ready to return to the industry full-time. Without Ivan, I still didn't know how I would begin to feel capable. Ivan had been my business partner and my biggest fan. He built me up when I felt insecure in business. He made me feel competent and confident. So how was I going to move forward without him? I had relied on him.

Ultimately, in October 2006, I accepted a full-time position in the San Francisco Bay Area. I purchased a condominium in Danville, California, with a loan against the equity of my home in Oregon. I was finally ready to take on the demands—physically, mentally, and emotionally—without Ivan. I thought I was over my grief. I had no idea the impact work would have on me.

In the early months of my new job, I put my head down and powered through the work. I traveled back and forth at least one weekend a month to take care of the Oregon property. It was overwhelming, having to learn what had changed in the industry in the three years since our retirement, managing the volume of emails, attending numerous meetings, and dealing with staff who were struggling in their own jobs.

I felt needed, but I didn't feel confident. It was as if I was catching up with everyone else, but I couldn't ask my peers for help. If I did, they'd know my secret—they'd know what I knew about myself—that I was incompetent. That need to not let others know I was struggling undermined my work relationships, and several of my peers did not care for me. By keeping myself at a distance, I created an environment at work that allowed me to work alone—with no partner, no support, no balance—but with a continued sense of inadequacy.

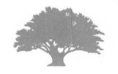

Chapter 48

Relationships

In addition to my attempt to return to the workforce, I also tried entering a new relationship. My counselor often used an expression with me when she talked about the person I was seeing. She said I was simply trying to "fill the shoes at the door." I thought I understood what she meant at the time, that I was looking for someone to love. I was. I was also looking for someone to replace Ivan.

I wanted to find someone just like Ivan—someone who would care for me the way he did, someone who was strong, smart, and independent—just like him. But I wasn't thinking about what I needed. I wasn't trying to find someone who was right for me. She felt that I simply wanted a man to fill the empty shoes Ivan had left. She was right. I was trying to find someone, anyone, who would return my world to what it had once been—someone to end the loneliness.

I met several men over the first couple of years following Ivan's death. My girls did not care for any of them, as they saw through the men I thought could fill Ivan's shoes. They could see that these men were not what I really needed or wanted. Each one was self-centered, demanding, or uncomfortable with my family. I didn't see it at the time, or at least I tried not to see it. Instead, I thought of Ivan—his likes, his mannerisms, his good points and his bad. I thought I could find someone who would carry on where he and I had left off. I suppressed any thoughts that I might never find that certain someone.

I often would lay awake at night, feeling an overwhelming sense of gloom. I was failing at this part of my life too. I felt empty as I compared each person against Ivan and the relationship we'd had. Ultimately, I ended each relationship. I couldn't seem to find the right person who would make me laugh and feel loved again.

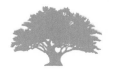

Chapter 49

Ditto

Shortly after Ivan's death, Purcy was attacked by a raccoon. She lost a portion of her ear and remained hospitalized for several days. As a result of the attack, the vet recommended that I consider giving her to a family in town since Purcy had always been used to being outdoors prior to our move to Oregon. Her love of the outdoors and my worry for her safety made the decision

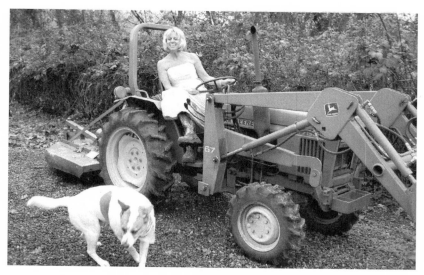

Ditto and me posing for our Christmas card photo – 2005

sad but necessary. In mid-2007, I found a loving family with kids, and they took Purcy to their home, where she could play and enjoy her life as a cat.

Thankfully, I still had Ditto as my loyal and loving companion. After Ivan's death, Ditto became my new partner. She followed me wherever I went, and I didn't go anywhere without her. She traveled back and forth with me from California to Oregon. When I cut the grass in the pasture, Ditto trotted behind the tractor at a safe distance. The pasture typically took six hours to cut, and after several rounds on the brush hog, Ditto would lay under a nearby tree and wait for me to finish.

Ditto loved music, and when I turned up the stereo in our living room and played certain songs, she would prance, like a horse, over to me. We would then dance around the room, with Ditto zigzagging in and out of my legs. It was hysterical to see her get so happy when the music was turned up loud. It signaled to her that we were going to have fun. And so, we would dance around the room: me with my dated, disco moves and Ditto prancing on all fours in and out of my legs as I moved. She was my companion; she made me smile with her human-like style; she comforted me when I cried.

During one of our weekend trips to the Oregon home, I was awoken around 1:00 a.m. by odd sounds coming from the back

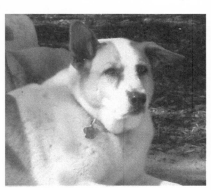

Ditto – 2006

room off the bedroom. As I turned on the light and got out of bed to investigate, I noticed Ditto was not asleep on the end of the bed as usual. I turned on the light in the back room and found her desperately banging her head into the corner, as if she were trying to get out of the room. I pulled her away from the wall, and she fell into my arms, panting and shaking. She did not try to get up, but lay there, sprawled out on the floor.

Frantic, I called a neighbor, and he immediately came over and helped me carry Ditto to the car. We raced her to the emergency vet, about forty-five minutes into town, and they took Ditto into the back room on a gurney. While I waited in the waiting room, I worried about what might be wrong. I remembered that she had held her back leg oddly the previous day, and I thought she had injured it in some way. There were no other signs of illness, so my mind scanned through a series of scenes that had occurred over the past few days, hoping to put the puzzle together. It was no use. I could not figure out what might be wrong, and my anxiety grew. I needed Ditto. She was my lifeline and my connection to Ivan and the memories we once shared. She was my companion and my joy. The thought of something being seriously wrong with her was unimaginable. My heart pounded, but I tried to calm myself as the clock ticked off the minutes.

After about forty-five minutes, the vet asked me to come to the back room so I could be with Ditto. When I entered the sterile surgical room, Ditto was lying on the stainless steel table with IV lines attached to her leg. She was restrained by white cloth straps, but she was still and didn't attempt to get up. She looked over at me as I entered the room and smiled, her eyes clearly acknowledging me. I stroked her side while the vet informed me that Ditto's spleen had burst. They could not save her.

Those words slammed into my head. I could not believe she was being taken from me. I needed her to stay and not die. As tears ran down my face, the vet gently told me that they could keep her on an IV for a while, but they needed my permission to inject the sedative that would end her life.

I openly began to sob. I did not want her to go. I wanted to lift her up and take her back home with me. Ditto looked up at me, listening to me cry. I could not look into her eyes. Those eyes wanted to know what was wrong. And they wanted to console me. How cruel life was to take such a loving companion from me and destroy my only source of joy.

I felt weak as I lifted Ditto's shoulders and held her in my arms as the vet carefully injected the medicine that would end her life. Her eyes smiled as she gazed up at me, and then they turned dark and empty. I was alone. It was only three years since I'd lost Ivan, and I was devastated. There would be no prancing dog, no dancing to loud music in the middle of the night, no more watching her sit under the large oak tree while I mowed the pasture, and no more long walks together. Only an overwhelming sense of emptiness remained.

As I returned to California from that horrific weekend and tried to focus on work, I struggled with the overwhelming sadness I felt for the loss of Ditto. I thought of life's crazy twists and turns. I thought about the coincidence that Ditto's spleen had ruptured—just like Ivan's. I tried to make sense of this additional loss and wondered what my life would become without her.

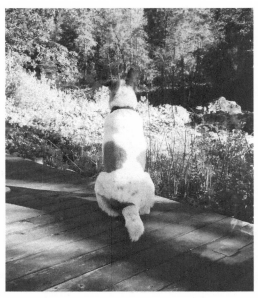

Ditto staring out across the river,
as she often did

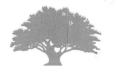

Chapter 50

Movement

Five years after losing Ivan, in December 2009, I decided to sell both my Oregon and Danville homes in preparation for a move to San Diego with the man I'd been seeing for the past two years. While I continued to focus on building a relationship that would replace the strong marriage I'd had with Ivan, I unintentionally sacrificed my assets in exchange for doing what this new man wanted. Trying to please him, the decision to sell would ultimately lead to significant financial loss.

The sale of my homes occurred during another downturn in the housing market. Both homes had dropped in value, but I took the biggest hit with the Danville sale because I'd purchased that property when the market was high. Although the sale took only four weeks, the damage to my finances was drastic. Because the value of my Danville home plummeted, I had to fund the balance of the bank loan in order to sell it.

That financial loss played over and over in my mind, causing me many sleepless nights, long after escrow closed. *What would Ivan think? Would he be appalled by the choices I am making in this new relationship? Would he be shocked by my need to be loved so much that I've been willing to sacrifice almost everything we built together?* In my heart, I knew I had not acted responsibly, and I began to admit to myself that Ivan would have been extremely disappointed in me. After all, I was disappointed in me. This single decision significantly reduced my assets—the very assets I was trying to rebuild and restore.

The following month, Oregon sold. Again, escrow closed quickly—in just three weeks. Although I didn't take a financial hit with the sale of this home, I lost several items of personal property because of additional decisions I made with my new love.

In just one weekend, I had to pack and move everything out of my fully furnished large home, workshop, and guest house. As my new love and I walked through the house, looking at my furniture and personal belongings, he pointed at each item and gave me instructions about what to sell, donate, or discard. Pleasing him seemed more important than preserving my belongings—even if it meant leaving everything behind.

I continued to have the nagging thought, *What would Ivan think?* Unfortunately, my desire to find happiness compelled me to give up much of my past life with Ivan and continue to move forward with this current relationship.

Ivan and I had never talked about what life would be like without him. He never shared his feelings and thoughts about my life after his death. After all, we were busy fighting the health sharks that had been circling us. To speak about life after his death would have been an admission of the fate that neither of us wanted to think about or face.

I refused to disclose to anyone, including my new love, the depth of sorrow I was feeling as I rushed to close the chapters in my life that related to Ivan and the decisions I'd made soon after his death. How could I tell this man about my reservations? I needed to pretend we were building something new together, and I hoped the emptiness I tried to deny would fade as we built new memories to replace those feelings. I was wrong.

The relationship ended a month later, in May 2010. I blamed him for the loss of so many precious memories and personal items. However, that was unfair. The truth was that I did not stand up for myself or for what I wanted—or needed. I had intentionally tried to clear my attachment to the past. He was simply my excuse as I attempted to run from my pain. Deep down, I was heartbroken that the Oregon property had become a place of sorrow and heartbreak, rather than a source of happiness in our retirement. It had not become what Ivan and I intended. We thought it was the perfect home for our retirement years, but without Ivan, I couldn't hold on to that vision. The blame for letting go of our home and our possessions belonged to me. I was the one responsible for the lost artifacts that had been a part of my life with Ivan.

To make matters worse, I ultimately lost some of the items I'd planned to keep. In the move from the storage unit, where I held my remaining personal property, several boxes were lost by the moving company. This was another reminder of my irresponsible actions and wrong decisions. Pictures and other valuables were lost. Once again, I had betrayed Ivan and our dreams together—and there was no way to ever get them back. I couldn't seem to do what was necessary to make Ivan proud; I was failing him and myself.

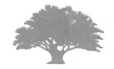

Chapter 51

"We" to "Me"

In September 2010, I purchased a home in San Diego. It was four months after ending my relationship with my boyfriend, and I was excited to start a life in a new place. However, in October 2010, my employer asked me to move to Hawaii to begin working there in December of that year. After I accepted the job in Hawaii, the company allowed me to travel back and forth once a month to San Diego to take care of my home.

Although the work in Hawaii only lasted a year, this move allowed me to create better working relationships because up to this point I had struggled in the workplace emotionally. I was grateful for the opportunity. As a result of my experience as a widow, with all of the challenges I faced, during my time in Hawaii I began to see more clearly who I had become: a woman who understood the value of people in my life, a woman who no longer worried about how people viewed me, and a woman who understood that the quality of my interactions with others was based on my opinion of myself and my perception of who I thought I was expected to be.

After I left Hawaii in 2012 and returned home to San Diego, I was given a new position within the company and continued to improve my interactions with both my staff and my peers. I no longer avoided people or felt compelled to hide my emotions. Having spent a significant amount of time dealing with my grief, I was more open with my coworkers. I began to gain confidence in myself and my abilities as my team and I executed various projects successfully. My work was not going unnoticed, and the accolades I received only helped to build my confidence even more.

I was changing emotionally, and I felt it. My grief from the loss of my business partner was diminishing. I loved being around friends and family, and I also loved pampering myself. I celebrated sunsets by taking time to stop and stare at them whenever I could. I created a ritual at my home that required my guests to stop whatever they were doing and join me in my toast to the sunset. It took only three to five minutes to stop, walk outside, stare off into the horizon, and watch the orange glow gradually sink below the ocean's edge as we raised a glass of whatever suited each person and toasted to the blessing of the sunset. It was worth it every time.

This new learning about myself was a direct result of my experience as a caregiver—learning to express my emotions rather than hide them in order to protect others, or even to protect myself. I embraced people, even those who did not care for me, and considered them all angels who were holding up a mirror for me to see what they saw. This approach helped me seek a greater understanding of myself, as well as those around me. I tried to understand more about was going on in other people's lives, so I could better understand what might be contributing to their approach to our interactions. This, then, allowed me to maintain a sense of peace with myself.

All of these changes occurred through subtle moments that took place over time. Eventually though, I began to see myself as a confident individual rather than just Ivan's partner. I began to see that I was capable of significant accomplishments without him at my side. As I started to acknowledge the person I'd become, I stopped trying to be someone else, I stopped making decisions that were better for someone else, and I stopped trying to find Ivan in everything I did or in the people I met. I was able to let go of the "we" to become "me," which was a key discovery that came out of my experience as a widow and learning to live without my life partner.

As I reflected on these changes, I found it interesting that my grief counselor had told me it would take five to seven years for me to resolve most of my grief. At the time, I had scoffed at that idea. Yet, there I was eight years later, finding my way on my own, no longer defined by my grief. It turned out that she had been right after all. Hawaii had allowed me to begin a fresh start without the baggage of the past, and the sale of my home in Oregon allowed me to release the connection to my life with Ivan.

By 2013, as I began to feel "me" more, I started to look at everything differently. I still felt Ivan in the places I went or in the things I did, but the feeling was of his memory—not about whether I was pleasing him or failing him through what I was doing. Instead, I began to feel comfortable that *I was doing what I wanted to do and it was for me.*

I felt the peace inside growing stronger and stronger as I became clearer about being "me." Since Ivan passed away, this was the first time I felt confidence, happiness, and peacefulness constantly. After nine years of walking backward, looking over my shoulder at the past, trying to make the present and future match those memories, I was able to stop that and move forward. It had been nine years of poor relationship choices, bad financial decisions, and running away from friends and family, as well as from my emotions, but I finally felt at home inside my skin.

The discovery of "me" gave me another gift as well. I no longer felt that I needed to be forgiven by Ivan or others for the outcome of his health. I forgave myself and let go of the feeling that I had been responsible for Ivan's death. I realized that my perception of my childhood led me to hold on to feelings of failure and a sense of inadequacy. I also recognized that any perceived failure was simply an emotion that I created. There had been no way for me to create a different outcome. Finally, and most importantly, the discovery of "me" helped me to understand that Ivan's silence toward me in his final days was his way of handling his own thoughts and feelings about his outcome and not about his disappointment in me. I now know, in the end, it turned out I couldn't save Ivan, but I was able to save myself.

Epilogue

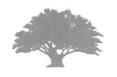

Chapter 52

Forgotten but Not Missed

When I finished writing this story and reflected on the numerous times I experienced Ivan's health issues, I remembered one particular, close personal friend who was always there for me. Her name is Jean. I am blessed to have several people in my life that I consider close friends, and I adore each and every one of them, but during this time in my life, Jean stood out as a confidant.

Vince and I worked at the same company and qualified for a top sales performers trip back in 1982. It was at this conference that I met his wife, Jean, and we became instant friends. Vince had become a close friend of Ivan's as well, and over the years of our marriage, we spent numerous occasions with the two of them. They joined us on a couple of family vacations, and we took several trips together. When they bought a home in Grants Pass, Oregon, we stayed with them as we searched for our future home in Oregon.

It was Jean whom I called when we got the news that Ivan had cancer, while we were traveling to our new home in Oregon. It was Jean whom I called when I stood outside the USF hospital in San Francisco after I had just been told Ivan had a 40 percent chance of survival. After we started our treatment process in Oregon, it was Jean who called me almost weekly, if not daily, to check up on me and talk to me about what I was feeling. She was a practicing marriage, family, and child counselor, and I trusted her implicitly with many of my emotions.

As I look back, I find it curious that I still felt alone, forlorn, and often desolate during Ivan's illness and my responsibilities as his caregiver when Jean was there for me whenever I needed her. I'm not sure why I chose not to remember that Jean was a source of comfort and a sounding board. I suspect it is because of the way I felt throughout our ordeal, rather than anything Jean said or did. I believe that despite her welcoming and loving style, I could not shake the feelings of inadequacy and failure, and so I did not talk to her about the emotions I kept hidden from everyone, including Jean.

In hindsight, there were lots of people who were present and who tried to help me during Ivan's illness, but I did not notice them. I was so focused on my own pain, on trying to make up for my inadequacies, on trying to control the outcome, and on saving Ivan that it was just too hard to turn to others for support, to open Pandora's Box, and to feel my emotions.

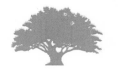

Chapter 53

Lucky

In retrospect, I see the painful descent Ivan and I entered into together from the time of his diagnosis in July to his death the following March. That eight-month descent was followed by an additional nine years of painful moments, as I journeyed alone through the grief process.

I wonder though...

If I had not run away from my emotions, not felt that I needed to pretend to be strong, not held on to the past, might I have moved through this time in my life with more ease?

Maybe...

But I believe in the statement, "I am exactly where I am supposed to be." Life and God placed me on this path for a reason, and I can now accept that.

There were a couple of coincidences that I was never able to fully explain, yet I believe they were significant parts of God's plan. The date and time of Ivan's death, 3.26, was one of them. Since he read the Bible daily before his illness, I looked at the Bible for a potential passage to provide meaning and found the Book of Job 3:26. "I am not at ease, neither am I quiet, neither have I rest; but trouble cometh."

Commentary about this passage indicated that in this chapter, Job's conflict began. Job was in great prosperity and peace when

Satan was permitted to touch his body and afflict it in the most grievous and distressing manner. But this turned out to be Job's triumph because through it all he never denounced God, and he accepted what was happening to him as part of God's plan. I believe Ivan also accepted God's plan for him, and ultimately, he clearly "let go and let God." The date and time of Ivan's death was a message to me that this was the triumph of Divine Grace in Ivan's life and Satan's ultimate defeat.

Ditto's spleen issue, like Ivan's, was another coincidence that I could not explain. Although I knew Ivan's slip and fall on the rocks had led to the rupture of his spleen, I was not aware of any injury to Ditto or an illness that would have caused her spleen to burst. I am left to wonder why her health situation mirrored Ivan's, but again, I believe it was a message to me: that I also needed to accept God's plan for me.

Finally, I will never know why Ivan did not choose to speak to me in his final days. As the reality of his prognosis set in, he may have been frustrated and bitter with his body, he may have been angry with me as the messenger of his fate, or he simply may have been sad, or completely exhausted from trying to fight for so long, and unable to talk to me about how he was feeling. I realize there are some things I will never completely understand, but I am okay with this fact today, knowing that through it all, God was with us.

Today, I consider myself lucky—lucky for the people who came into my life after Ivan passed away and for the people who are in my life now, lucky for meeting people who were selfish and negative, as much as for the people who were loving and constructive, for they all helped me to see what I was doing to destroy myself. They helped me to understand the pain I was creating by holding on to the memory of a man who could no longer hold me in his arms, by holding on to the dreams we had once planned together. All of these "angels" helped me to learn who I was and who I had

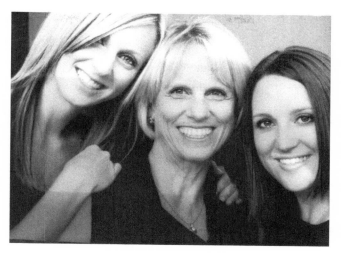

Sara, me and Alison – 2010

become. Oddly enough, I felt reborn. Yet, little did they realize the impact they'd had on my life.

Work became a source of joy and contentment until my retirement in 2018. I came to value the people I worked with from 2013 to 2018 and felt confident at work, as I regained my passion to help others in their careers.

I met with a priest and reconciled my disconnect from God and my faith, and I now appreciate the magic of angels and the Lord in my life.

Alison and Kye now have three children and live in the San Francisco Bay Area, and Sara and her two children live in San Diego. My mother is ninety-one years old, and my sister and brother continue to help her as needed.

In July 2012, I responded to a friend request on Facebook, only to discover it was an old high school friend, Bruce. He had learned that I was a widow and located me on Facebook. On August 12, 2012, I met Bruce, and we revisited our history and started dating. Bruce is a retired policeman from Arizona.

Bruce and I married on February 14, 2015, and we moved to our new home in Southern Oregon in July 2018. Coincidentally,

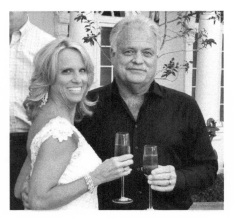

Bruce and me on our wedding day –
February 14, 2015

our home is on a river about forty-five minutes from my former home. He adores my family, and they love and admire him as well.

We have a new puppy, a Bernese mountain dog named Orie (after Oregon). She is not Ditto, and I'm not trying to make her be that beautiful dog. Orie is a loving, gregarious pet who has brought new joy into my life with Bruce, and she is a special dog on her own.

Today, Bruce and I spend our days working together around our property, spending time with friends and family, training Orie, and fulfilling the dreams we have together as retirees.

Some Final Thoughts
for Caregivers

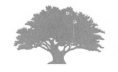

Chapter 54

Angel Messages

As I mentioned at the beginning, no matter how unique each person's story may be about being a caregiver, the feelings concerning expectations of a caregiver and all of the "shoulds" imposed by ourselves and others, real or imagined, are remarkably similar.

My journey to forgive and accept myself occurred over time. This did not happen through a single event or person. This process was slow and required me to conduct an honest reflection of my emotions and behaviors before I could pardon myself for the perceived mistakes in Ivan's care, as well as his death. Like grieving, it couldn't be rushed.

In writing *Take Care of Ivan,* I was able to look back and see myself as a caregiver through a different lens than when I was in the midst of my husband's illness. I was able to see that I truly did do my best to *Take Care of Ivan.* And I realized that as I wrote my story about being a caregiver, angels delivered healing messages to me that were meant for me to offer to you. Maybe one—or all—of these whispers is meant for you:

• *Angel Message:* **Remember that your past can influence your present and the decisions you make or avoid.**

I was able to recognize that the influence of my background, childhood, and other personal experiences that preceded my caregiver role set the stage for my emotional reactions, interpretations, and struggles. I realized I had placed self-imposed burdens on myself regarding Ivan's care that resulted in feelings of guilt and inadequacy when things did not go well. I had let my past control how I accepted the events as a caregiver.

- *Angel Message:* **Don't let society dictate how you should act.**

I let the influence of society's impression of how a caregiver should act dictate the way I shielded my true emotions. I did not open up to my children, as well as to others around me, for fear of reprisal for the negative thoughts I had about Ivan's illness and the struggle I experienced with his care.

- *Angel Message:* **Everyone who comes into your life is an angel.**

While I was in the role of caregiver, I did not trust people, or ask for or accept help. I thought I could do everything myself and needed to prove that I could. I worried about pleasing others—the selfish ones as well as the loving people. I later learned to embrace all of the people who came into my life.

- *Angel Message:* **Be kind and don't judge yourself.**

During my time as a caregiver, I beat myself up on several occasions when things went wrong with Ivan's illness. After his death, I wanted desperately to make good decisions, to do things right and redeem myself because I felt responsible for Ivan's death. I also found the caregiver role demanding, with many ups and downs that tested my strength. At times, I struggled to maintain my composure and manage the various tasks I needed to perform to support Ivan's well-being. There were times when I hated the things I had to do, and I felt weary and exhausted.

- *Angel Message:* **Give up trying to control things.**

  Ivan had an expression, "God has a plan, and He's on time, and so let go and let God." Whether you believe in God, a higher power, or just yourself, this message is about giving up control. I tried to control everything within my role as caregiver, including Ivan's health outcome. Control somehow made me feel confident, and the harsh reality I learned is that I control very little around me, except how I feel about things.

- *Angel Message:* **Keep the honest, authentic, and vulnerable you visible to the world.**

  When I cared for Ivan, I was extremely guarded with my emotions. I thought I needed to appear strong and not let anyone know how scared I really was about his illness, about being alone in the country, and about trying to manage the hundreds of tasks I needed to do for him. I did not want people to see my true self, so I faked a smile every time I interacted with anyone.

- *Angel Message:* **Seek to understand the motives for your behaviors.**

  I engaged in several self-destructive behaviors, especially after Ivan passed away. I was not conscious of the motives behind my actions, but many of my actions were destructive nonetheless (at least not in my best interests emotionally, physically, or financially). It took several years of self-reflection before I realized what I had been doing.

  As a caregiver, you have the opportunity to grow into a new, more expansive and compassionate version of you. While you are in the midst of caring for others you may not recognize this, but when you believe this is part of the process, you will see your transformation sooner and embrace those moments of opportunity.

Through these angel messages, I know now that I was exactly where I was supposed to be as a caregiver, and you are too. And regardless of where you are at this very moment, a significant, traumatic event, such as caring for a loved one or losing a loved one, will not only change you—it will transform you. It did me!

Acknowledgments

Thank you to the supremely talented editor Donna Mazzitelli for shepherding *Take Care of Ivan* through the editing process with grace, passion, wisdom, and emotional support.

Thank you to Susie Schaefer and Polly Letofsky at My Word Publishing for keeping me on track and providing invaluable advice.

Thank you to Donna Cunningham for the intuitive ability to design the perfect book cover.

Thank you to all the friends and family who lived through the days before, during, and after the writing of this memoir.

Thank you to my two daughters for always being there for me.

And a very special, loving thank you to my husband, Bruce, who provided the strength and courage I needed at the right time, every time, when I wasn't sure whether I could or should write this book.

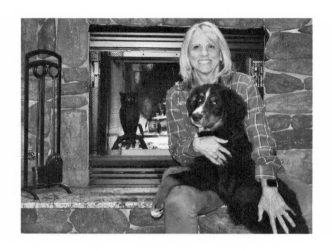

About The Author

Suzanne Anest has forty-four years' experience within the healthcare industry. Without the benefit of a college degree, she achieved financial success, as well as managed several highly effective teams. Suzanne was one of the first female sales representatives in the group insurance industry in the 1970s. She was a member of the Top Sales Producers Forum several years in a row before transitioning into management.

Suzanne owned and operated her own benefits consulting firm for ten years, before retiring in 2002. After the death of her husband Ivan, she returned to work in 2006 and worked for a large healthcare firm, continuing her business career for another twelve years before retiring for good in 2018.

Suzanne was born in California, where her immediate family still resides today. She has two daughters and five grandchildren, and she loves spending time with each of them. Suzanne has a diverse passion for various hobbies, including sewing, beading, and fishing, and she enjoys working around her home, doing landscaping and managing household repairs.

Suzanne wrote *Take Care of Ivan* with the intention of helping other caregivers manage their trials and expectations. Today, Suzanne lives in Oregon beside a river with her husband, Bruce, and their dog, Orie.